Psychosis, Spirit Possession, and Child Sexual Abuse

T0383765

This distinctive volume examines the psychological claims of spirit possession and psychosis as they are linked to child sexual abuse, intimate partner violence, and poor mental health.

In the context of both clinical complaints and community-based determinants, this book uses Jungian and Fanonian theory, political history, and case study analysis to explore the systems at work in projecting internalized traumas of colonialism and personal powerlessness onto a scapegoated demonic presence affecting victims/survivors of sexual violence. It focuses on populations of the global south but is relevant to victims of oppression worldwide, considering the personal unconscious and cultural complexes that influence a sense of being overtaken and controlled by supernatural or intrapsychic forces or a desire to be.

Psychosis, Spirit Possession, and Child Sexual Abuse offers an alternative framework for understanding mental processes that lead to symptoms such as auditory or visual hallucinations that often get misdiagnosed and mistreated. This is important reading for practitioners and scholars of depth psychology and is of keen interest to academics in the fields of foreign and cultural studies, as well as students and researchers in sociology, religion, or anthropology.

Hazel Da Breo, PhD, is a Canadian scholar-practitioner of Grenadian birth and Indigenous ancestry. She has co-authored three academic texts on Child Sexual Abuse in the Caribbean, co-authored a book chapter on Feminist Narrative Research, and authored numerous articles for peer-reviewed journals on a wide range of psychological subjects including museums as sites of colonial oppression. Having worked as a consultant to various United Nations agencies over the last two decades, she currently directs a multi-year project for Global Affairs Canada concerning the sexual abuse of children under the age of five. Hazel is a graduate of a master's degree program in Depth Psychology (Pacifica Graduate Institute), Adult Education (Yorkville University), and Art History (York University). Her PhD in Psychotherapeutic Counselling is from the Open International University. She is the co-founder of an NGO, Sweet Water Foundation: Research and Treatment Institute and a Professor of Psychology at St. George's University. Her current research interests center on the Neuroscience of Trauma and the Philosophy of Cultural Psychiatry.

'This unique and pioneering work embarks on a bold exploration of the complex intersections between mental health, spiritual experiences, and the trauma of child sexual abuse. Hazel Da Breo's insights and compassionate approach offer hope and understanding for those navigating the aftermath of profound trauma. Arising from decades long work as a psychologist and heavily influenced by phenomenology and spirituality, her work is not only an academic and therapeutic achievement but also offers deeply moving narratives that honor the lived experiences of survivors. As a Co-Founder of an organization dedicated to combating violence against women and girls as an issue of structural discrimination, I believe Da Breo's contribution to our understanding of trauma and the paths to recovery is significant. I believe that this book will be an invaluable resource for therapists, survivors, scholars, activists, and anyone committed to the deep work of healing and liberation.'

Jaspreet Singh, *JD, Co-Founder, ICAAD*

'Page by page Hazel Da Breo in *Psychosis, Spirit Possession, and Child Sexual Abuse: A Jungian, Depth and Liberation Psychology Perspective*, challenges our view of trauma or better said our view of an objective reality. She argues our heuristic scientific training as therapists detaches and distances us from our child abuse patients' experience and our own humanity. It denigrates insights of thinkers such as Jung and Fanon, Sufi Emmanuel Vaughan-Lee, and Jean-Martin Charcot. She, as a fellow traveler among them, is an unapologetic phenomenologist. She places the lived experience of our patients, from the banal and quotidian to the worrisome and terrifying to the pleasurable and numinous, at the core of how we can help resolve their suffering. She presents us with accounts of ten children, each of whom jumps to life in her telling. They have experienced terrible acute experiences and chronic dysregulating quotidian experiences. The chronic experiences are what I call the in-between times. The in-between times are the child's reiterated moment-by-moment growth distorting, benign or growth enhancing experiences with others that fill the child's life between the acute events. It is repetition of the banal experiences of the child in the in-between times that sculpt how the child sees the world and her way of being in the world. Simultaneously, as Da Breo gets us inside the child to see how the child experiences the world, rather than how we would see the child's world, she raises our thinking to the possibility of psychosis as a cultural manifestation of spirit possession. And while admitting that the full range of specific factors that affect children of specific groups is unknown, she presses us to consider Indigenous practices, colonization, social adversity, racism, exclusion, city vs. rural living along with other factors as playing a role. Da Breo's book will bring you back to the essence of doing the work we love. Even those of you who view children's trauma as an objective outcome of distorted brain processes, Da Breo's writing will expand how you think and work with your traumatized patients.'

Ed Tronick, *PhD, Professor of Psychiatry and Pediatrics, University of Massachusetts Chan Medical School*

Psychosis, Spirit Possession, and Child Sexual Abuse

A Jungian, Depth, and Liberation Psychology Perspective

Hazel Da Breo

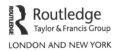
Routledge
Taylor & Francis Group

LONDON AND NEW YORK

Designed cover image: Sea Lungs by Asher Mains (2015)

First published 2025
by Routledge
4 Park Square, Milton Park, Abingdon, Oxon OX14 4RN

and by Routledge
605 Third Avenue, New York, NY 10158

Routledge is an imprint of the Taylor & Francis Group, an informa business

© 2025 Hazel Da Breo

British Library Cataloguing-in-Publication Data
A catalogue record for this book is available from the British Library

Library of Congress Cataloging-in-Publication Data
Names: Da Breo, Hazel, author.
Title: Psychosis, spirit possession and child sexual abuse : a Jungian, depth and liberation psychology perspective / Hazel Da Breo.
Description: Abingdon, Oxon ; New York, NY : Routledge, 2025. | Includes bibliographical references and index. |
Identifiers: LCCN 2024027763 (print) | LCCN 2024027764 (ebook) | ISBN 9781032122120 (hardback) | ISBN 9781032122113 (paperback) | ISBN 9781003223603 (ebook)
Subjects: LCSH: Sexually abused children--Mental health. | Sexually abused children--Rehabilitation. | Spirit possession--Psychological aspects. | Psychoses--Religous aspects.
Classification: LCC RJ507.S49 D22 2025 (print) | LCC RJ507.S49 (ebook) |
DDC 618.92/85836--dc23/eng/20240729
LC record available at https://lccn.loc.gov/2024027763
LC ebook record available at https://lccn.loc.gov/2024027764

ISBN: 978-1-032-12212-0 (hbk)
ISBN: 978-1-032-12211-3 (pbk)
ISBN: 978-1-003-22360-3 (ebk)

DOI: 10.4324/9781003223603

Typeset in Times New Roman
by KnowledgeWorks Global Ltd.

Contents

Acknowledgments

I am indebted to many works of scholarship spanning the disciplines of psychology, psychotherapy, anthropology, religion, and art. I am especially grateful for the scholarship I undertook at Pacifica Graduate Institute, where I learned a profoundly different way of looking at the world; it is the Depth tradition that I acknowledge for my main intellectual formation, but I recognize all of the many teachers who guided my lifelong learning in psychology. This includes the original team of human development specialists I worked with in the early days of my UN consultancies in the Caribbean and Latin American Region: Roberta Clarke, Alex Vega, John Waters, and Cherise Adjodha. I also acknowledge my first team of writing colleagues, Adele D. Jones, Ena Trotman-Jemmott, and Priya Maharaj of Huddersfield University, from whom I acquired more wisdom than any book-learning could bestow. I thank June Douglas, Chair of the Humanities and Social Sciences at St. George's University, who spiritedly encouraged my teaching, research, and writing efforts. Thank you to Antonia McDonald, Associate Dean of Graduate Studies, St. George's University, for her nurturing spirit and clarity of mind. Thank you to Damian Greaves, Associate Dean, School of Arts and Sciences, St. George's University, for his very powerful expression of support.

Great gratitude to Cherise Adjodha. Beyond her critical insight and phenomenal intellectual scope, I am most deeply grateful for her friendship and emotional accompaniment on this journey. Cherise would not allow any limitations to shackle my creativity during the hyper-obsessive phases of my writing, lived with me in the village of my mind, and allowed me to cry. Not everybody can catch the therapist's tears. Linda J. Butler, Josef Peidelstein, and Frederick Prack, thank you for turning up this lifetime. As I consider Toronto my spiritual home, so do I consider you three to be my spiritual family, my soul-keepers. Etric Lyons, thank you for our conversations on psychoacoustics. Yes, the river must flow. To Manon Beset, Katie Randall, and the rest of the production team at Routledge Taylor Francis, you were phenomenally patient and pleasant through this book-making process. Thank you so much for your professionalism and kindness. At the level of scholarly input I offer gratitude to Dr. Doris Keens-Douglas, M.D., Psychiatrist, Ministry of Health, Mt. Gay Mental Health Centre, St. George's Grenada; to Dr. Gerard Hutchinson, M.D.

Professor of Psychiatry, University of the West Indies, Mona, Trinidad and Tobago; and to my research assistant at St. George's University, Mjolnier Messiah.

Dr. Timothy Cook, my physician in Toronto, made a powerful contribution to my writing quite unbeknownst to him. Along with saving my life when I was unwell, it is his very beingness as a professor, doctor of functional, integrative medicine, yogi, medical anthropologist, PTSD specialist due to his 20-year military career, and practitioner of the contemplative sciences that has left an indelible impression; he literally manifests all that a healer can be.

Gratitude to my ancestors, known and unknown, for the sure-footedness with which they have collectively guided me, often over terrain that I would have resisted having to cross. As for my family and children, they are in my hands as I write, in my eyes when I see, and in my lungs as I draw breath. I cannot thank my children, all six of them, for anything less than giving me life.

Most importantly, I thank my clients, the most rigorous teachers of all, who forced me to abandon all the theories I had memorized and reconstruct them again using my own mind. It is through the practice that I have most richly learned and grown.

Land Acknowledgment

I acknowledge the original caretakers and storytellers of the land where I was born, the Kalinago people of Grenada and the Caribbean of whom I am a proud descendant. I commit to honoring their determination to remain free and tending to our environments, psychologies, and stories. I acknowledge the original nations of the territory where my mother later situated me, Toronto. These include the Anishabeg, Chippewa, Haudenosaunee, Huron-Wendat, the Mississauga of the Credit, and many diverse First Nations, Inuit, and Metis. I am grateful for the privilege of gathering in your spaces, and I commit to sharing responsibility for protecting children and the other vulnerable inhabitants of the earth.

Foreword

Cherise Adjodha

I am deeply honored to be writing the foreword to Dr. Hazel Da Breo's first monograph. I have worked in the field of human development for the past 25 years with some of the world's leading development agencies, and I have seen much that is deeply troubling and indeed heartbreaking. This eloquently written and deeply felt work from Hazel has renewed my faith in what we can reimagine and enact in the way of addressing child sexual abuse and in healing those affected.

I met Hazel over a decade ago when I worked with the United Nations Development Fund for Women (UNIFEM), now known as UN Women. As many of us in these fields of work know, whilst we have some successes, which are not to be overlooked, we are often in the broadest sense, feeling what seems an uphill battle against the darker sides of our human nature. How many programs and interventions have we done? How many times have we found ourselves no less than begging for support to heal our fractured societies?

I have worked with Hazel on regional batterer intervention programs, education on adolescent sexual and reproductive health and rights, policy, and legislative reform for the protection of the rights of children and the prevention of violence, and other interventions. Hazel's range of expertise ensured the provision of insight into the human condition, which was deeply unique and essential.

I had the privilege, I realized, of working with someone who not only understood the importance of the individual but also the importance of understanding their experience "in relation". That is, in relation to other practitioners, their families, institutions, communities, justice systems, and even to the surrounding physical environs within which we exist together.

Over the years, I have journeyed with Hazel both as a colleague and friend and have seen the remarkable work she has done as practitioner, teacher and as herself an evolving student. Ever in the pursuit of more understanding, and not maintaining the stasis of a fixed mind.

You will see this demonstrated throughout *this text*, as Hazel explores the experiences and circumstances of victims, perpetrators, families, institutions, fellow practitioners, and others. Revealed are insights into the microcosm and the macrocosm of our social worlds, and how they interconnect, interrelate, and interdepend on each other, for their perpetuation. You will see strength and fragility and will understand better the intersections of our shared lived experiences.

As you journey through, you will find yourself asking: What must we do differently now? What must we transform? What is healing? What is true justice? In fact, at times you will ask, what is real? What is the fabric of the reality that we collectively share, and how can we heal its fractures?

While common approaches to having been "wronged", to having witnessed the effects of trauma, are to pathologize and dehumanize, often not only perpetrators, but also victims, Hazel has a keen awareness that, addressing what causes sexual violence, what creates this behavior, also requires healing, not simply punishment. Therefore, we must address our individual and collective humanity.

This book gives us the opportunity to do this, and compels us to consider: What can be more revealing of the vulnerability and complexities of our human experience, than to look into the trauma of an innocent child? What patience, what wisdom and enduring strength must we have, to help a mind and body that is yet still forming, to make sense of the most painful experiences?

In her capacity as a profoundly accomplished, intelligent, and discerning healer, through her writing Hazel also invites us to ask and seek to understand: What of the perpetrator? What cultivated their behavior? What of their lived experiences? What of those who stood still and watched and did nothing? What of those who deny, and who victimize further those who have been robbed of their innocence, of their sovereignty and indeed of their ability to love themselves? Robbed of the desire to be loved, and to be alive. What of our own pain? Our own trauma? Our own desire to heal?

Hazel gives insight into our hidden and sometimes even visible ghosts, the seemingly fantastical psychological phenomena that can be our lived experiences of darkness. The experiences we deny, pathologize and therefore continue to cultivate. We are reminded that trauma has a past, a present and a future within which we are all conscripted to participate, lest we intervene in this here and now. *This book* invites us to support the healing of the moment and to look at the pain of trauma with a wide and heart-centered lens.

Yes, this may seem daunting, but perhaps what is most important about this work, is that in addition to its eloquent yet difficult to "hear" honesty, it will ignite your courage, not your despair. The true essence of this work, and why it ignites my faith in our ability to heal ourselves and each other, is that Hazel does guide us through and out, to our liberation.

Psychosis, Sprit Possession and Child Sexual Abuse demonstrates that in our willingness to confront unimaginable pain, the willingness to work together from our multiple perspectives, and through our devotion to healing and protecting our children, we can not only survive, but we can flourish.

In its true essence *this work* is an invitation to explore, to experience, to inquire and to act. This work is about the now, and about our future. With deepest gratitude to Hazel, and to you the reader, for journeying through this work.

sincerely,

Cherise Adjodha

Yara

The Opening

Yara sat on the sofa in the space where her father's hand patted between himself and her Mum. Knees together, ankles crossed, private school pleats crisply pressed into her skirt, the scent of the rain forest still rose wild from Yara's skin. Fixing her gaze on the icy lake only separated from us by the Distillery District's red brick warehouses at the point where the city's spine touched Lakeshore, she answered softly to each question in the same manner; "I wouldn't say" she responded, "I wouldn't know". But in Yara's eyes, her knowing was infinite and certain when she gifted us with a direct stare. In stark contrast to her parents' agitation, as they hurled descriptions of the transformation that Yara underwent at dusk when she writhed and twisted in her bed, uttering sounds of insanity and connection with beings unseen and unheard by any others, Yara now sat composed, calm, profoundly spirited indeed but in full command of the energies that moved her. If the gods possessed her, as her parents claimed, it would seem that Yara invited them in with purpose.

While I would offer a sound psychological response to the symptoms of psychosis that Yara's parents tumbled over each other to describe, the colleague beside me, the Reverend Dr. Andrade, would offer the shamanic interpretation that was in keeping with his own cultural experiences and training. We weren't the same, psychologist and shaman, but neither of us was wrong. We each focused on the phenomena we observed, un-storying the false narratives and sifting away the muddy dramas foisted upon us by Mum and Dad. We differed only in our language of explanation but in spirit, we were essentially the same with Yara.

Yara's unfolding took years. Her parents had requested a duo of therapists: myself, a Caribbean Canadian woman, and Andrade, a Latin American man. Together, we worked softly and slowly, pulling at the iron-clad armor surrounding Yara, her parents, their stories, and the apparent intrusion of a dark and overwhelming psychic force that visited her under the shadow of night. As an author, I share this case with you much as it was revealed to us, just a little at a time. Andrade and I often felt ourselves stumble between whirlwinds of emotion, impenetrable silence, and continuously shifting realities. We waded through veiled truths, obscured facts, and intra-familial behaviors that sometimes manifested in direct contradiction to the established parental narrative. But we persevered. There was a child at risk, so we held on by the teeth.

Such is the work of psychotherapy; it is sometimes intensely mystifying but always a deeply rewarding process.

"Be careful when you cast out your demons that you don't throw away the best of yourself."

Friedrich Nietzsche, Thus Spake Zarathustra.
https://www.gutenberg.org/files/1998/1998-h/1998-h.htm

Preface

As a psychotherapist working for several decades on issues of child sexual abuse, I have witnessed and confronted the deep complexities of the human condition. As a professor of psychology, I have similarly had to confront the academic ways in which child abuse traumas are typically categorized, explained, and diagnosed, sometimes being at odds with the lived realities of individuals.

As my work evolved, it became clear to me that traumas caused by childhood sexual abuse often give rise to symptoms that may be diagnosed as psychosis or as spirit possession, depending upon the worldview of the attending practitioner. I have found that the ontological position of the practitioner, in this regard, is critical to understanding how trauma is interpreted, understood, and addressed as a bio-psycho-social and cultural phenomenon. I began my practice in the late 1970s; since then, I have gathered hundreds of accounts from clinical and field engagement with individuals from the diverse populations inhabiting Toronto and the Caribbean and Latin American Region, which are my homes. Therefore, my views on psychosis are a direct result of my experiences as a psychotherapist working in a multi-cultural, multi-ethnic context and within a range of social and economic environments.

The effects of child sexual abuse (CSA) vary in many ways; still, it is generally agreed that the impact is lifelong and that the depth of trauma experienced can have repercussions reaching far beyond what can be easily addressed or explained. The focus of this book is on the intersections between CSA and interpretations of the symptoms of that trauma as either psychosis or spirit possession, depending upon the views of the clinicians at hand.

Bourgeois et al. (2021) make strong linkages between child sexual abuse and the early onset of psychosis symptoms, and the World Health Organization refers to acute psychotic episodes as "exacting some of the largest tolls conceivable on human beings… being particularly lethal in low-income settings" (WHO/PAHO, 2018). The American Psychological Association writes that Child Sexual Abuse (CSA) and other Adverse Childhood Experiences (ACEs) may lead to death. Yet, the precise developmental course or experience of psychosis following CSA remains unknown. In addressing these deep unknowns, I have developed a practitioner's viewpoint, which has led me to the field of phenomenology. As a phenomenologist, I am committed to directly examining the multiple, subjective complexities of human experience rather than, or ahead of, theoretical notions of objective reality. Phenomenologists are typically obsessed with the concrete, to the point of distrusting theoretical hypotheses and accounts.

> Description, for the phenomenologist, is … to return repeatedly to the phenom- enon Itself so that it may show itself in ever more profound, richer and more subtle ways. This repetitive return is the disciplined and self-critical hermeneu- tic circle. Therefore, the description is not opposed to interpretation, but the interpretation is required to remain intrinsically descriptive.
>
> (Brooks, 2015, p. 32)

The hermeneutic circle described by Brooke is derived from the Greek word *heuriskein*, which means to discover or find. In the 1990s, Clark Moustakas founded the "heuristic research" process for psychology, and it has since been used in numerous diverse fields, from nursing to math and computer programming. In heuristic research, the researcher's self is present throughout and is responsible for describing their direct and personal engagement with the phenomenon under investigation. The heuristic approach thus proves uniquely demanding of research- ers and their readers, as it deliberately keeps away from the detached, anonymous, authoritative style of many writers in psychology. A certain vulnerability thus en- velopes the fold for researchers and readers when work of this nature is engaged.

In relation to child abuse trauma, I place the lived experiences of victims at the center of all that emerges as a direct pathway to the resolution of their suffering. Researchers working within an autoethnographic framework typically declare this positionality like myself. This helps us come to terms with our ontological perspec- tive and situate both inherent and constructed social contexts as important. Posi- tionality resists data depersonalization and understands research as being "rooted in stories lived and told" (Clandinin & Connolly, 2000, p. 20). As Mc Cormack et al. (2020) wrote, "The self of the researcher is a substantive, constituent fabric in the epistemological tapestry" (p. 75).

My journey as a phenomenologist began in the Buddhist community, where phenomenology derives its force from the systematic development of an essential discipline, meditation. This journey has now come full circle in my study of Sufism and Islam, which solidified itself during a 2019 trip to Jerusalem, where I presented to the International Congress in Spirituality and Psychiatry, hosted by the World Psychiatric Association, on this very subject of child sexual abuse, spirit posses- sion, and psychosis.

It was on a quiet suburban street in Richmond Hill, Ontario, where I lived for over 25 years, that I found an unassuming Theravada Buddhist temple where like- minded Canadians gathered to practice meditation under the tutelage of the resi- dent monks. This was my first direct experience with formal phenomenology. We aimed to learn how to lessen suffering through observing consciousness and the melting away of troubling emotion, or *néantiser*, as Sartre would say. As I battled an ongoing personal *nigredo* in the following years, I took several trips to Thailand, where I practiced with the Forest Monks of Chiang Mai in their monasteries, caves, and jungles. There in the wild, natural world, where icy rivers rushed by at our feet and breezes carried the sound of raucous macaws, there was a sense that the mist-laden mountains themselves nurtured our benevolence, that the pneuma of all beings, sentient or material, was vital and pure. I felt my senses sharpen considerably, and I learned to concentrate fast. Personal transformation was impossible to resist, but the most precious outcome was my new, pervasive sense of being free, a perpetual personal objective.

Freedom in the Buddhist tradition can be understood as a life without suffering, a mindful way of inhabiting the world. As I drove away from Wat Dhammamongkol in Bangkok at the end of my last stay, the head monk at the time, Pra Maha Supon, called out to me, "Stay in the Forest!". This was not meant in the physical sense, of course, but as a reminder of the strength, resilience, and freedom of the forest we carry inside.

Back home in Toronto, a new internship at the Zen Buddhist Temple provided an entry into the discipline of Psychotherapy, where I would continue to analyze the relationality of experience and the constitution of meaningfulness through meditation and clinical practice. My intention to help myself and others observe the very formation of suffering deepened through a constant return "from talk and opinions to the things themselves, questioning them as they are themselves given, and setting aside all prejudices alien to them" (Szanto, 2014, p. 35). In other words, learning to remain free of bias, misinterpretation, and subjective reductionism. Later on, during formal academic study, I realized that the three psychiatrists whose ideas most influenced my vocation as a psychologist were also phenomenologists: R.D. Laing, Franz Fanon, and C.G. Jung. Phenomenology has become my professional, explanatory method and a personal orientation for me as a scholar-practitioner, my natural disposition. Existential phenomenology, in particular, offers a depth of possibilities for describing the multifaceted lived experiences of the clientele I have engaged since I have found myself working largely with victims of various kinds of trauma and also because an extraordinary personal investment is demanded of those working with this population and in this vein. In practice, as in the writing of this book, I aim to bracket my very life choices in phenomenology, to take a clear, concrete, and unblinkered view of what I perceive well before I begin to place theoretical notions upon those perceptions.

Romanyshyn wrote that Phenomenology and depth psychology are therapeutics of humanity's modern psychological life. Fundamentally, a successful psychology praxis not only takes in this theoretical position writ large, but in each day's practice, it also takes on the sacred task of a refreshed and sustained commitment to liberating every patient from their individual mental and psychic oppression. As Buber wrote concerning the "psychosis of war" and the joint responsibilities of *raison d'état* and *raison d'être*, "In the commandment 'Thou shalt not kill' can also be heard the commandment "Thou shalt not kill the soul of your people" (Buber, p. 225). Psychology has a liberatory purpose, as Ignatio Martín-Baró and Paolo Freire proposed. In this text, where the specific phenomenon of psychosis as a scientific, psychiatric condition is discussed, I also discuss the medical, psychological, spiritual, and cultural systems of belief that often cause the suffering of people with psychosis not to be alleviated and set free, but instead to be misperceived, weaponized, and augmented.

While I do not attempt to provide an exhaustive technical description of these terms as their theorists do a much more effective job than I do, phenomenology, hermeneutics, and case study analysis, under the umbrella of the Depth, Jungian, and Liberation Psychologies, are the tools I use for guiding my foray into the relationships between child abuse, psychosis, and spirit possession. Where I write of the arousal of the dark feminine, or what has been called spirit possession in the specific cases that I describe, this dark feminine arises, not as an abnormal psychology but as an almost predictable, almost *desirable* defense mechanism against the shattering of the human mind when it has been subjected to chronic abuse or very adverse childhood experiences.

I intend to hold to a strictly psychological understanding of the psychic turmoil I have witnessed in my practice. As Hillman wrote, understanding is perhaps the most operational of all Jung's concepts, as he places his approach within the tradition of psychologies of *understanding* rather than psychologies that are explanatory, descriptive, or medical in the narrow sense. Where I have heard psychic states named either psychotic or demonic, it has usually been a factor of the prejudices of practitioners. I would like to state my dependence upon ethnography, medical anthropology, religion, and psychology in my process. In the end, this text is an interdisciplinary offering.

C.G. Jung recognized that his approach to transcultural psychiatry was essentially phenomenological (Abramovitch & Kirmayer, 2003), and I have naturally followed his path from phenomenology toward hermeneutics, or hermeneutic phenomenology which, as I have mentioned before, is a theory and methodology of interpretation that tries to get to the *a priori* essence of the thing under examination. It informs the most indigenous of indigenous psychologies, being absolutely committed to the subject's own phenomena or the client's real existence and pretheoretical, primordial experience. Case study follows as the most powerful method known to practitioners in various fields for investigating and explaining contemporary phenomena in real-life contexts and for adding richness to the information presented. In cases involving psychotic breakdowns in children and young adults, where the contexts out of which the breakdowns come are unknown or unclear to professionals though critically important, the joint framework of phenomenology, hermeneutics, and case study analysis has scaffolded my aim to illuminate the complexities inherent in each individual's lifeworld or *Lebenswelt* (Husserl, 1969). This framework allows me to "see straight" and to arrive at my understanding of the relationships between child sexual abuse, psychosis, and what is referred to as spirit or demonic possession in many traditional cultures, including the ones into which I was born. I aim for a holistic view of the process via which a mind breaks and scatters itself and earns itself a diagnosis of either schizophrenia or possession.

Here, I do not attempt to present a comprehensive understanding of the psychoses, nor do I describe my personal treatment methodologies. Instead, I attempt to explain how symptoms of child sexual abuse trauma may manifest interchangeably as psychosis or as spirit possession, depending on the ontological understanding, language, and experience of the practitioners (not the patients).

Even though there is now a vast literature on all aspects of child abuse, I yet believe that this particular form of human tragedy escapes a distinctive voice. Finally, along with aiming to understand the action of psychotic breakdown from the actor's point of view, not simply as a result of external forces but primarily as a result of the creation and organization of the subject's understandings, the discourse within their mind, I question what exists in our collective cultures that renders children so everlastingly at risk of sexual violence, mental breakdown, and psychic possession. At the same time, too many knowing adults stand by, apparently complicit in grievous harm and insufficiently concerned about the implications, thereby leaving statistics to continue to rise. Statistics include the staggering financial costs of mending the mental health diseases of victims who have broken down.

I contemplate the oppression of children and other vulnerable populations, and I also reflect upon the oppression of psychology itself and the frequent failure of the discipline to meet its liberatory purpose. The term Depth Psychology was first coined by Eugen Bleuler in 1914 in reference to the science of the unconscious and the patterns and dynamics of motivation and the mind. Depth psychology seeks knowledge of the deep layers underlying behavioral and cognitive processes. Bleuler, along with Freud, Jung, and Alfred Adler, are all considered Depth Psychology's foundations. Jungian psychology introduced the idea of the collective unconscious, in which all lives and minds are enmeshed in common wisdoms, which are played out in symbols, myths, and patterned storytelling. Jung introduced archetypes as primordial elements of the collective unconscious, including instinctual and religious or metaphysical energies. Liberation Psychology joins Depth and Jungian Psychology as guiding philosophies of my personal praxis, a joint approach to making men and women more fully and authentically human. Just as Paolo Freire's 1970s call to make education accountable to social need was beginning to resound globally, Ignatio Martín-Baró also pioneered Liberation Theology and then Liberation Psychology, which concerns itself with individuals and groups who are marginalized and oppressed, with the intention to identify the biological, psychological, and social agents of their oppression.

Liberation psychology focuses on ethnically diverse and indigenous communities, guiding individual choice away from passive helplessness and depression toward the courage and power necessary to overthrow "invalidating environments", inclusive of motivated engagement within a new therapeutic life space. Liberation psychology also recognizes that the problems of the oppressed are reflective of cognitive distortions inherent in the oppressor's mind as well, an idea reflected by Franz Fanon when he discussed the impact of violence upon the perpetrator and the evolution of cultural unconsciousness in general. Fanon proposed urgently developing a new pedagogy for psychology and its treatments with the decolonization of oppressive states of being as the end goal. Considering processes of individuation or self-actualization on both individual and collective levels, as Depth and Jungian psychologies do, Fanon described the moment or process of enlightenment as "the moment of awakening … when the oppressed find the oppressors out…and begin to believe in themselves" (Freire, 1970, p. 64). "This, then", Freire wrote, "is the great humanistic and historical task of the oppressed: to liberate themselves and their oppressors as well" (1970, p. 44). Through these contemplations, I have also focused on the role of the psychologist and on the overall discipline of psychology, not only in terms of social justice approaches to mental health in communities in general but also in terms of the very framing of disease and the language of our framing, which from the start will either lead individual patients on the path to personal freedom or keep them suffocated within the darkness of mental and spiritual confusion. In criticism of the ongoing Westernization of psychology, Fanon's biographer, Hussein Abdilahi Bulhan, wrote that "psychology as an organized discipline…is Eurocentric through and through". C.G. Jung, too, had flung his net far and wide to ensure that Depth Psychology not be seen as a solely European construct, and more recently, Sunan Fernando wrote that "the psychiatric diagnostic process allows the discipline of psychiatry to function in such a way that racist ideology is absorbed and applied in a scientific guise".

Psychology being a discipline of interiority, we in the Depth tradition view illness from the inside, focusing on the client's lived reality rather than from a collection of signs that manifest externally and which are left to the experience of practitioners to interpret. Jung referred to his psychological inquiry as setting out upon a *Mare Ignotum* (unknown sea), and R.D. Laing (1964) wrote that the practice of psychiatry too often relies exclusively upon the analysis of medical records and pieces of paper rather than the lived realities and behaviors of the person, in the clinic as well as in life.

Regarding spirit possession, I approach it in like manner as I would do psychology because a much more fluid, pluralistic, and embodied notion of selfhood is indicated in psychic phenomena than the DSM currently affords. In 1992, the American Psychiatric Association's Diagnostic and Statistical Manual of Mental Disorders introduced possession as a defined, carefully described mental disorder. While giving recognition to this form of suffering and placing it in the hands of psychologists where the phenomenon rightly belongs, it also pathologized what is normal and even predictable in some cases of early childhood trauma, stigmatizing and demonizing understandings of the professed demonic.

This has not been an easy book to write, nor, I suspect, will it be easy to read. Wherever I have spoken publicly on the subjects of sexual violence and child abuse, some have become visibly agitated and left the room. Many have approached me afterward to say they felt I had recounted their own personal story with eerie precision. This is whether I have spoken on home ground or in territories as far away as Israel, Thailand, or the hinterlands of Guyana. On the one hand, diverse global contexts are crucial in their differences, but on the other hand, a child is a child.

Lombardi et al. (2019) wrote that "all forms of psychosis must not be lumped together indiscriminately: every case should be evaluated separately to determine the actual possibility of … treatment being beneficial" (p. 83). Although Bourgeois also indicated that the developmental course of psychosis following CSA remains unknown, I hope that the collection of case histories in this text, gathered over decades, will help to illuminate this developmental course, the shadowy terrain where numerous opportunities to identify and treat child victims of sexual abuse may be missed. Jungian, Depth, and Liberation psychologies inform the lens through which I offer you this journey. Although I write with a full focus on these people's inner, lived realities, that is, with a psychological view, I acknowledge that I do not escape intersectionality. I am deeply concerned with the particularities of these cultures where alarming rates of child abuse, psychosis, and complex spiritual possessions continue to rise without there being a felt understanding of the interconnectedness between the diverse elements, much less a remedy for the traumas.

If you have experienced abuse as a child, my love to you.

Note that all identifying features of the people and situations that I describe in this text have been significantly altered to protect the privacies of individuals, groups, and communities.

References

Abramovitch, H., & Kirmayer, L. (2003). The relevance of Jungian psychology for cultural psychiatry. *Transcultural Psychiatry*, *40*(2), 55–163. https://doi.org/10.1177/1363461503402001

Bourgeois, C., Lecomte, T., McDuff, P., & Daigneault, I. (2021). Child sexual abuse and age at onset of psychotic disorders: A matched-cohort study: L'âge d'apparition des troubles psychotiques chez les victimes d'agression sexuelle à l'enfance: Une étude prospective de cohortes appariées. *Canadian Journal of Psychiatry. Revue Canadienne de Psychiatrie*, *66*(6), 569–576. https://doi.org/10.1177/0706743720970853

Brooks, J. (2015). *Learning from the Lifeworld*. The British Psychological Society. https://www.bps.org.uk/psychologist/learning-lifeworld

Freire, P. (1970) *Pedagogy of the Oppressed 30th Anniversary Edition*. (Trans). Bloomsbury Academic.

Husserl, E. (1969). *Ideas: General Introduction to Pure Phenomenology (F. Kersten, Trans.)* Martinus Nijhhoff Publishers.

Laing, R.D. (1964) *Sanity, Madness and the Family: Families of Schizophrenics*. Penguin Books.

Lombardi, R., Rinaldi, L., & Thanopulos, S. (Eds.). (2019). *Psychoanalysis of the Psychoses: Current Developments in Theory and Practice*. Routledge.

Szanto, T. (2014). Social phenomenology: Husserl, intersubjectivity, and collective intentionality. *International Journal of Philosophical Studies*, *22*(2), 296–301. https://doi.org/10.1080/09672559.2014.896624

World Health Organization/Pan American Health Organization [WHO/PAHO]. (2018). *The Burden of Mental Disorders in the Region of the Americas*. https://iris.paho.org/bitstream/handle/10665.2/49578/9789275120286_eng.pdf

Introduction

Introduction

Increase in Child Mental Health Disorders: Child Abuse Psychosis (CAP)

Several reports describe an increase in mental health problems among children (Cuellar, 2015; Holland, 2016; Budde et al., 2023). During the COVID-19 pandemic, an alarming youth mental health crisis came to the fore, signaled in America by the American Academy of Pediatrics and the U.S. Surgeon General, who issued an advisory on the urgency of need among children and teens (2021). However, youth mental illness was already on the rise well before the pandemic, with an increase of 40% in high school students, more than one in three disclosing persistent feelings of sadness and hopelessness. Between 2009 and 2019 in America, one in five had contemplated suicide in the same time frame (Centers of Disease Control and Prevention [CDC], 2023). The National Institute of Mental Health (2010) believes that one in five children has a mental health disorder in any given year, and worst, 17.4% of children between the ages of 2–8, have a diagnosed mental health condition (Cree et al., 2018). One-half of mental disorders have an onset before the age of 14 years, and finally, in America, more attention is now paid to the mental health of preschool-age children (Danielson et al., 2018; Curtin & Heron, 2019; CDC, 2020).

Notably, NHIS data from 2017 to 2018 for children and adolescents aged 3–17 years showed that boys were more likely than girls to have seen a mental health professional during the past 12 months and that parents of boys were more likely to have spoken with a doctor about a child's emotional or behavioral problems (CDC, 2020). Along with these statistics indicating a gendered discrepancy around care provision, UNICEF reported (2019) that 15% of adolescents from low and middle-income countries have attempted suicide. This points to a racialized discrepancy in which Black children had the highest prevalence of behavioral or conduct problems (Meek & Gilliam, 2016; Rafa, 2018). Because evidence has shown that racial bias can result in certain behaviors among Black children being incorrectly interpreted as disruptive, this finding might represent

DOI: 10.4324/9781003223603-1

overdiagnoses or misdiagnoses that are masking other forms of mental distress among Black children. Considering this book's focus on child sexual abuse and its manifestation in Child Abuse Psychosis (CAP, a term I have coined to describe the psychosis-like symptoms arising specifically from child sexual abuse), these statistics put Black female children from low and middle-income countries in a particularly high-risk bracket of incorrect or insufficient psychiatric diagnosis and care.

The word psychosis was first used in the mid-80s in Germany, by Karl Friedrich Canstall and Ernst Baron Von Feuchtersleben. In 1899, Emil Kraeplin, in Germany, acknowledged that 5% of future schizophrenics had already presented symptoms in childhood. By 1906, the Italian psychiatrist Sante de Sanctis identified very early dementia as a form of child psychosis. Eugen Bleuler (Moskowitz & Heim,1911) similarly acknowledged schizophrenia occurring in childhood, and in 1933, H. W. Potter began to use the term "infantile psychosis", leading to the isolation of four different types of child psychoses: Autistic, Symbiotic, Deficit-based, and Pscyhormomies. However, a diagnosis of psychosis was not actively applied to children until the late 1980s, when Paul Moreau de Tours recognized the possible presence of symptoms before puberty (Houzel, 2005). In this text, I propose the term Child Abuse Psychosis (CAP) to refer to the mental breakdown that ensues as a specific result of child sexual abuse.

The demand for mental health services for child and youth populations is thus immense, or ought to be immense, but when these children come from lower socioeconomic communities, their parents (often comprising a single mother alone) are hard-pressed to find the time or money to take them into extended therapeutic care. Emotional wounds go untreated until they erupt volcanically, at significant financial and social cost to society. According to the CDC, the estimated lifetime cost of rape is $122,461 (U.S.) per victim, or a population economic burden of nearly 3.1 trillion over victims' lifetimes (Peterson et al., 2017). In 2019, the World Health Organization launched its Special Initiative for Mental Health, which would advocate for universal mental health care coverage due to such rising incidents and their financial burden. Still, this coverage is unlikely to reach the child populations of the global south.

Additionally, if the mental health issues become severe, as in the case of child abuse psychosis, and if the client manifests symptoms co-morbid with rage, aggression, and conduct disorders, the young clients may find themselves in conflict with the law and thus twice removed from adequate, sensitive care. The ten case studies presented in this text are exclusively focused on descriptions of the experience of psychosis from the points of view of the clients themselves. However, the more significant impacts on society are also made clear.

Incest, sexual molestation, child abuse, domestic violence, and human trafficking have all made headlines in a variety of news and social media in the last few decades. It is incredibly heart-breaking to watch the humanitarian crises currently befalling the children of Haiti, Palestine, the Sudan and elsewhere, along with migratory caravans of undocumented peoples crossing borders all over the world with vulnerable children in tow. It is especially daunting to imagine the level of mental health care that they and their families will need in the future.

In 1983, the film *Something About Amelia* provided the first sensitive treatment of incest for a national audience. In 1985, *The Color Purple* did the same. We have become more aware of international rings of child pornography and pedophilia, not carried out by monsters in the closet but on an institutional level. In Hollywood, 2018, we saw Bill Crosby charged and imprisoned for sexual assault. In 2011, Jeffery Epstein was charged with the predatory trafficking of young women, and in 2012 his female partner Ghislaine Maxwell emerged as one of the first women charged with helping her male partner groom underage girls for sexual exploitation. In Toronto, Paul Bernardo, dubbed the "Schoolgirl Killer", pulled off a series of rapes in Scarborough between 1987 and 1990, in which his then-wife, Karla Homolka, was responsible for luring victims into her husband's grasp, including her own younger sister. We thus have been forced to contest the archetypal image of the female as perpetually nurturing and life-giving and to recognize that any sex or gender may perpetrate the abuse of children. In the Caribbean, it was found that while violence is mainly (but not exclusively) perpetrated by males against females, many children have reported that they received their first beating at the hands of their own mothers (Jones et al., 2014). As a six-year client recently shared with me, "Have you ever seen blood on you, Miss? I did. I saw some blood on me. My mother burst my head, and blood came out of my head through my mouth. More than one time".

Culture is normally described as having to do with religion, art, cuisine, language, and dress, or what amounts to the four cultural attitudes defined by Joseph Henderson (Kimbles, 2003): social, religious, aesthetic, and philosophic. But as Fanny Brewster very poignantly adds (2020), culture is also defined by child-rearing practices.

In a recent Netflix docuseries, *Monique Olivier: Accessory to Evil* (2023), the serial abduction, rape, and murder of ten adolescent girls by Michel Fourniret over the span of 17 years in France is chronicled as "exceptionally sadistic", "abominable", and "indescribable". Before they married, Michel wrote to Monique from prison, where he was incarcerated for previous sexual assaults. He confessed both his past actions and future intentions to Monique, writing, "I want to deflower a virgin. When my penis has pierced a virgin's womb, I will be a man like any other". Once released and married to Monique, she played an active role as an accomplice to murder, with some experts believing that she only came alive through the crimes of her husband. Commentators referred to both man and wife as a satanic, assassin couple.

In the final analysis, as the narrator underlines, it was not the police that stopped them. Not a lawyer, not a judge, or the police. It was one brave little girl who managed to break free and run away to tell her tale. In this text, the ten case studies that I describe illuminate both the victimization and the bravery of the children involved. Along the path to maturity and individuation, human beings may find themselves alternately victimized and triumphant in multitudes of complex ways.

Child Sexual Abuse, however, represents perhaps the most severe type of victimization, with little chance of complete survival and healing without targeted psychological assistance.

In 2017, the #MeToo movement and its sisterhood of survivors was catapulted into international fame, becoming a global rallying cry against sexual violence on an unprecedented scale and making its founder, Tarana Burke, an iconic activist. Today, TikTok carries numerous stories from women all over the world of the sexual abuses they suffered at the hands of perpetrators, who are generally older family members, both male and female.

Child abuse is a major problem and not just something that happens in marginalized communities. It is the almost total power of adults over children, the result of a distorted power complex that is inextricably linked to patriarchy and colonialism. However, not only the patriarchy is to blame. As Cunningham (1986) wrote, perpetrators of sexual violence are very much locked into the traditional masculinist expectations of dominance. Yet these men often fail to meet social expectations of dominance or even of adequacy, failing at school, at work, in relationships, and otherwise. They feel powerless in a multiplicity of ways, so children and other vulnerable groups, therefore, become their only means for recovering that power. In other words, while this is a major societal problem, it is also an individual psychological problem.

A much deeper understanding of how cultures and communities are constructed is called for, of the role that human biology plays in the development and manifestation of trauma, how individual personalities are formed, and how the political governance or cultures of child-serving institutions themselves all come into play. In other words, a deep psychological understanding of these myriad meaning-making mechanisms of victims, perpetrators, bystanders, and institutional orientations is called for.

This text offers an understanding of the role of patriarchy and cultural complexes in sexual violence against women and children, which includes the tendency for those who feel powerless (male or female) to perpetrate acts of violence upon groups or individuals who are perceived to hold less power, regardless of their sex or gender. This text also looks at individual psychologies and deconstructs the relationship between child sexual abuse, psychosis, and possession by so-called demonic forces. While addressing the psychosocial trajectory of victims of sexual violence from relative good health to mental breakdown, this text, more importantly, speaks to the potential for both girls and boys to harness the tremendous power of the feminine to overcome chaos and not only survive but to move very powerfully toward magnificence.

Child Abuse and Psychosis

Along with reports of increased mental health problems among children and youth, an increasing number of studies are demonstrating an association between childhood abuse and psychosis (Fischer et al., 2011). Beginning with Freud and others who developed their theories that adult psychopathology is rooted in adverse childhood experiences (1890s), a considerable body of literature has emerged linking Adverse Childhood Experiences (ACEs) with a range of mental health disorders and negative social outcomes in later life. Despite this powerful trope of evidence, the linkages between childhood sexual abuse and psychosis remain largely overlooked, with the exception of a few large-scale population-based studies (Janssen et al., 2004; Whitfield et al., 2005; Bebbington et al., 2011).

One limitation to studies like these is that CSA remains underreported, particularly in cases of incest, in cases involving very young children, in cultures where silencing is enforced, and where bystanders are not mobilized. In other words, as stratospheric as the known statistics are, we have yet to realize that CSA is very largely under-reported.

Nevertheless, there is a considerable weight of evidence linking childhood sexual and physical abuse with psychosis. More specifically, childhood rape was significantly associated with visual, auditory, and tactile hallucinations.

These experiences include physical abuse by the main mother and father figures (usually but not necessarily the biological parents), sexual abuse by any adult or an individual at least five years older than the recipient, parental antipathy (hostility, rejection, or coldness), and emotional or physical neglect (Fischer et al., 2011).

A significant proportion of people develop psychosis in adulthood following all types of childhood abuse, including people diagnosed with schizophrenia, major depressive disorders, dissociative identity disorder, and post-traumatic stress disorder. Evidence suggests a causal relationship between childhood abuse and psychosis in adulthood (Manning & Stickley, 2009) and that early adversities may lead to psychological and biological changes that increase psychosis vulnerability (Janssen et al., 2003).

Regarding treatment protocols for victims of CAP, unless we get a reasonably clear picture of the underlying vulnerability, therapeutic endeavors risk being misguided. If a patient has had a traumatic experience that is followed by psychosis, there are completely different therapeutic implications than if the patient has long-standing vulnerabilities.

Failure to inquire about abusive experiences has been shown to be common among clinicians, but there is some movement toward making this part of all routine psychiatric assessments (Fischer et al., 2011). A considerable number of psychiatrists writing in the British Journal of Psychiatry (2008), criticized the lack of evaluative and classification skills among mental health practitioners working with psychosis. Furthermore, the majority of psychiatrists themselves also lack crucial skills and understanding of aspects of psychosis. In summary, psychosis remains a besieged citadel whose walls have not yet been breached by any practitioner. To this, I add that where CSA is indicated, no treatment approach will be fulsome without skilled expertise in healing from this very specific type of child abuse trauma.

The Catastrophic Interaction Hypothesis

The onset of psychosis can be a devastating and harrowing event in the life of a young person and their family particularly if their backgrounds include early chronic child abuse trauma. In this text, I do not pretend that all instances of child abuse culminate in psychosis; indeed, there is no simple cause-and-effect relationship between psychosis and any trauma. However, considering a complex array of biopsychosocial variables, the disruption to a person's developmental trajectory is nowhere seen to cause such ongoing emotional devastation as cases of child sexual trauma, whether resulting in psychosis or not.

Speaking of spirit possession ensuing from sex abuse trauma, I want to end this introductory segment with a brief mention of one of the ways in which C.G. Jung described possession, as it is instructive to the way I understand possession, too. First, it is noteworthy that Jung used this term to describe the dramatic "possession" of the entire nation of Germany by Hitler. Again, a similar situation is playing out in Gaza as I write. In history as well as in myth, there are numerous examples of whole groups, populations, and nations who follow a leader to perpetrate phenomenal harm or good. I address this further in the chapter on Bystander Mobilization in this text. Consider the Pied Piper, Dionysus, the Bacchae and Martin Luther King Jr. on the one hand, and Lord of the Flies along with Hitler and settler colonialism on the other. Examples abound in literature and life. From the first hypnotic word of the adult incest-abuser to their child victim, through the varied states of consciousness that befall families, communities, and cultures where silence in the face of gendered violence and oppression in all of its forms is normalized, there are many angles from which we can look at "possession" or "grooming". Considering all of these various angles, categorizing the emotional distress of child victims (as opposed to the mental states of their oppressors) as pathological or as a possession seems the most disingenuous angle of all. Yet, in this text, I do aim to take a systematic look at why some victims who have broken down are referred to as possessed, psychotic, or just plain mad.

Spirit possession may be seen as a good and desirable thing in different contexts. Today, as we witness many of the world's peoples rising up in support of the indigenous Maori of New Zealand and their fight for sovereignty, I have been taken with the inherent spiritual force displayed by women and children in particular. The Haka dance, incorporating fierce facial expressions with bulging eyes meant to intimidate opponents, stamping, and other gestures of stylized violence, are precisely the gestures that are likely to be ridiculed in other cultural contexts and mocked as a type of possession by evil or mischievous spirits. Suppose this is indeed a type of possession; in that case, it is a possession that is cried out for and embraced as the strength and endurance of ancestral spirits are sought to help individuals and communities through an apparently insurmountable difficulty. Many indigenous cultures nurture this type of relationship with the ancestral realm as with God, the saints, and the angels. Still, in the colonized West, such proud resistance has been exorcised from us and driven out along with our languages, religious beliefs, and methods of child-rearing, among so many other variables. In this discussion on child abuse psychosis, it is timely to take another look at this native tradition of calling for ancestral assistance. In fact, in the cases of Maddinks, Yara, and Bahira, we can see that the tradition has never left us but perhaps simply tunneled underground or into the collective unconscious, awaiting invocation by women, girls, and warriors. We will definitely see that those cases remaining unhealed represent victims who, unfortunately, had all personal and ancestral strength entirely drained out of them by their abusers and colonizing forces. We see that the rising of the "dark feminine", be it in a girl or a boy, and whether it is actually a helping energy rather than a harmful one, its manifestation may lead to a diagnosis of possession or psychosis rather than a valid mental health condition and result in us being subdued and institutionalized.

As both Fanon and Yara might, I hear this predicament as a voice of violated and abandoned children and nations, and we collectively urge all helping entities to never stop illuminating the dark corners of oppression, in whatever its forms and in whatever ways we can. For example, in 2022, the Guardian published an article in which the brutal rape of women and children is used by gangs as a weapon of war. Médecins Sans Frontières reported approximately 100 victims of rape per month at their clinic in the capital (*The Guardian*, Nov. 14, 2022).

In this text, please note that I have chosen to use the term "victim" instead of the mental health community's currently prescribed term of "survivor". It is a carefully considered choice, as while the trend is to move to the apparently more powerful assertion that one has survived the assaults of an abuser or abusers as immediately as possible, I argue that these terms exist on a continuum. The movement is a journey often comprising as many failures and setbacks as successes, and the path is not linear. By this, I mean that each individual who has experienced abuse may find themself sliding up and down the scale between victim and survivorhood throughout their lifespan, thus moving from powerful self-agency to sudden overwhelming flashbacks and fears. It is accepted that alcoholics never refer to themselves as recovered, always as "recovering". Similarly, people living with PTSD, their families, communities, and healers all know that despite the APA's total capacity of mental health intelligence and treatment approaches behind it, victims remain susceptible to triggers that may repeatedly propel them back into their trauma syndromes. I have found it to be similarly so for many victims of rape trauma. Note that PTSD is a diagnosis developed for soldiers of war, but that the second largest population of people living with PTSD is victims of child sexual abuse. I consider it, therefore, unkind to expect child abuse victims to rise to salvation ahead of patients with other psychiatric disabilities. I would rather hold space for individuals to assert in their own time when they feel themselves to have recovered or whether they still feel in need of the social and medical supports that are not always extended to those claiming recovery status and survivorhood. I believe it a disservice to belittle or truncate the very real, lived reality of the struggle to recover from child abuse trauma meaningfully.

References

Bebbington, P., Jonas, S., Kuipers, E., King, M., Cooper, C., Brugha, T., Meltzer, H., McManus, S., & Jenkins, R. (2011). Childhood sexual abuse and psychosis: Data from a cross-sectional national psychiatric survey in England. *British Journal of Psychiatry*, 199(1), 29–37. https://doi.org/10.1192/bjp.bp.110.083642

Brewster, F. (2020). *The Racial Complex: A Jungian Perspective in Culture and Race*. Routledge.

Budde, S., Walsh, W. A., Waters, J., Kacha-Ochana, A., & Irving, K. (2023). A Children's Advocacy Centre comprehensive initiative to increase engagement with children's mental health services. In A. St-Amand, P. Rimer, D. Nadeau, J. Herbert, & W. Walsh (Eds.), *Contemporary and Innovative Practices in Child and Youth Advocacy Centre Models* (1st ed., pp. 253–274). Presses de l'Université du Québec. https://doi.org/10.2307/jj.4032504.19

Centre for Disease Control and Prevention [CDC]. (2020). *Youth Risk Behavior Survey Data Summary & Trends Report 2009–2019*. Division of Adolescent and School Health. https://www.cdc.gov/healthyyouth/data/yrbs/pdf/YRBSDataSummaryTrendsReport2019-508.pdf

Center for Disease Control & Prevention [CDC]. (2023). *Data and Statistics on Children's Mental Health*. Children's Mental Health. https://www.cdc.gov/childrensmentalhealth/data.html

Cree, R. A., Bitsko, R. H., Robinson, L. R., Holbrook, J. R., Danielson, M. L., Smith, D. S., Kaminski, J. W., Kenney, M. K., & Peacock, G. (2018). Health care, family, and community factors associated with mental, behavioral, and developmental disorders and poverty among children aged 2–8 years—United States. *Morbidity and Mortality Weekly Report*, 67(5), 1377–1383. http://dx.doi.org/10.15585/mmwr.mm6509a1

Cuellar, A. (2015). Preventing and treating child mental health problems. *The Future of Children*, 25(1), 111–134. http://www.jstor.org/stable/43267765

Cunningham, D. (1986). *Healing Pluto Problems*. Weiser.

Curtin, S. C., & Heron, M. P. (2019). *Death rates due to suicide and homicide among persons aged 10–24: United States, 2000–2017* (352). Centers of Disease Control and Prevention [CDC]. https://www.cdc.gov/nchs/products/databriefs/db352.htm

Danielson, M. L., Bitsko, R. H., Ghandour, R. M., Holbrook, J. R., Kogan, M. D., & Blumberg, S. J. (2018). Prevalence of parent-reported ADHD diagnosis and associated treatment among U.S. children and adolescents, 2016. *Journal of Clinical Child & Adolescent Psychology*, 47(2), 199–212. https://doi.org/10.1080/15374416.2017.1417860

Fischer, P., Krueger, J. I., Greitemeyer, T., Vogrincic, C., Kastenmüller, A., Frey, D., Heene, M., Wicher, M., & Kainbacher, M. (2011). The bystander-effect: A meta-analytic review on bystander intervention in dangerous and non-dangerous emergencies. *Psychological Bulletin*, 137(4), 517–537. https://doi.org/10.1037/a0023304

Holland, D. (2016). College student stress and mental health: Examination of stigmatic views of mental health counseling. *Michigan Sociological Review*, 30, 16–43. http://www.jstor.org/stable/43940346

Houzel, D. (2005) *Invisible Boundaries: Psychosis and Autism in Children and Adolescents*. Routledge, https://doi.org/10.4324/9780429476235

Janssen, I., Krabbendam, L., Bak, M., Hanssen, M., Vollebergh, W., De Graaf, R., & Van Os, J. (2004). Childhood abuse as a risk factor for psychotic experiences. *Acta Psychiatrica Scandinavica*, 109(1), 38–45. https://doi.org/10.1046/j.0001-690x.2003.00217.x

Janssen, I., Bak, M., Krabbendam, L., Hanssen, M. (2004) Childhood abuse as a risk factor for psychotic experiences, February 2004, *Acta Psychiatrica Scandinavica 109*(1), 38–45. https://doi.org/10.1046/j.0001-690X.2003.00217.x

Jones, A. D., Jemmott, E. T., Maharaj, P. E., & Da Breo, H. (2014). An integrated systems model for preventing child sexual abuse. In: *An Integrated Systems Model for Preventing Child Sexual Abuse*. Palgrave Macmillan. https://doi.org/10.1057/9781137377661_1

Kimbles, S. (2003). Joe Henderson and the Cultural Unconscious. *The San Francisco Jung Institute Library Journal, 22*(2), 53–58. https://doi.org/10.1525/jung.1.2003.22.2.53

Manning, C., & Stickley, T. (2009). Childhood abuse and psychosis; a critical review of the literature. *Journal of Research in Nursing, 14*(6), 531–547. https://doi.org/10.1177/1744987109347045.

Meek, S. E., & Gilliam, W. S. (2016). Expulsion and suspension in early education are social justice. *National Academy of Medicine*. https://doi.org/10.31478/201610e

Moskowitz A, & Heim G. (2011). Eugen Bleuler's Dementia praecox or the group of schizophrenias (1911): A centenary appreciation and reconsideration. *Schizophr Bull. 37*, 471–479.

National Institute for Mental Health (2010) Statistics - National Institute of Mental Health (NIMH) (nih.gov) https:www.nih.gov/health/statistics.

Peterson, C., DeGue, S., Florence, C., & Lokey, C. N. (2017). Lifetime economic burden of rape among U.S. adults. *American Journal of Preventive Medicine, 52*(6), 691–701. https://doi.org/10.1016/j.amepre.2016.11.014

Rafa, A. (2018). *Suspension and Expulsion: What is the Issue and Why Does it Matter? Policy Snapshot*. Education Commission of the States. https://eric.ed.gov/?id=ED58150 0externalicon

The Guardian. (2022) 'Women's bodies weaponized': Haiti gangs use rape in spiraling violence | Haiti | *The Guardian.*

Whitfield, C., Dube, S., Felliti, V., Anda, R. (2005). Adverse childhood experiences and hallucinations, Pergamon, Child Abuse and Neglect. https: www./hearingvoicesusa.org/images/stories; https://doi.org/10.1016/j.chiabu.2005.01.004 (hearingvoicesusa.org)

Part I

Psychosis

Chapter 1

Carrie

Carrie was just shy of her 16th birthday when she walked into the city square and felt her brain slip out of her head and run onto the pavement, thick and poisonous as mercury. Something about the wide spaciousness of the urban setting caused her many fractured little parts to unstick and float off, looking for containment, but there were no boundaries to be found. At the end of the distance was a massive parking lot, beyond which the great lakes spread themselves wide, and the sky rolled away above, cold and unfeeling.

Carrie stood perfectly still, watching her mind slip further and further from her grasp. One tributary of her liquid senses ran into a crack in the sidewalk and disappeared below the ground. "I am subterranean", Carrie thought, "There I go". She struck a pose, as in a childhood game of Sly Fox, and vaguely wondered if she should even try to gather herself back together again or press her face into the earth and return herself to dust.

On the one hand, she experienced the slippage of her mind as a massive burden rolling off her shoulders, but on the other hand, she grieved its leaving. After a lifetime of perseverance, of pulling herself back together – her pajamas, her shame, the shutters on her windows, her bedsheets, her hidden parts – in this wide urban space, her center did not hold. She suddenly imagined the women from her village heading home after a long day of de-bushing the roadside, and declining Carrie's mother's invitation to sit down and rest for a while. "If we sit down now, we will drop asleep one time", they'd say. Likewise, as Carrie had stumbled across the skies on an Air Canada flight not two months before and exhaled for the first time that she could ever remember, she finally dropped completely apart.

"Wait", she said to her disappearing mind. "Wait". The pavement moved. It lurched and trundled forward like an escalator, heading for the dark-skinned lake in the far distance. "No, wait". Carrie pulled out of her freeze and flung her arms wide, grabbing for railings and barriers of any kind, but nothing. That evening, I met her hospitalized, courtesy of the passersby who witnessed the visible, public spectacle of her breakdown and dialed for help. Diagnosis: out-of-touch-with-reality, non-affective first-episode psychosis. "It's not me that you see", Carrie told them as they processed her admission. "I am not made of glass; you cannot see through me".

DOI: 10.4324/9781003223603-3

When she had arrived to safety in Canada, the state of hyper-vigilance in which she had lived, the high levels of adrenaline and cortisol that had fueled her for the last decade or so of her life, now reacted to Carrie's experience of physical safety by moving into such sudden recovery and recuperation that she collapsed altogether.

Psychiatry defines psychosis as a treatable medical condition that occurs due to a dysfunction of the brain, causing people to have difficulty separating false, personal experiences from reality (Compton & Broussard, 2009). It may co-occur with other mental health issues, such as mood disorders and Post Traumatic Stress Disorder (PTSD), and exists on a full continuum with schizophrenia at the most extreme end. Psychosis includes prodromal symptoms or early warning signs like changes in beliefs about self and others and self-harming or abusing substances. The continuum makes the experience unique for each person, ranging in duration, severity, and level of distress or function impairment. Symptoms generally include hallucinations and delusions or decreased energy and motivation.

Most lay people relate psychosis to the phenomenon of hearing voices. Still, according to Romme and Escher (2013), "The term psychosis is a mystification. We believe that calling hearing voices 'hallucinations', and unusual beliefs 'delusions', or to call both of these 'psychotic symptoms', is unjustified and harmful and that these terms handicap building a relationship with the person whom they hinder" (Romme & Escher, 2013, p. 1).

In Carrie's case, her prodromal symptoms of insomnia, mood swings, suspiciousness, paranoia, dropping out of social activities, and general anti-social behaviors had begun to develop when she was about nine years old, not being an early onset of psychosis but an early onset of sex with her father. Additionally, while her disorganized speech, disorganized behavior, and visual hallucinations were tangible signs of positive psychotic symptoms, these, too, had been with Carrie from the initiation of the incestuous relationship. This is what I introduce as Child Abuse Psychosis (CAP). The symptoms are often the same, but their origin is quite specific, and their treatment must also be quite specific.

In psychiatry, there is an increased indication that genes and neurodevelopmental abnormalities are less causal to psychosis and other psychiatric conditions than the complex interaction between those elements and environmental factors. Indeed, since 1977, the stress-vulnerability model was proposed by Zubin and Spring, which not only pointed to stressors like abuse as causal factors but emphasized protective factors in reducing vulnerability. Epigenetics also speaks to how lifestyles, environments, and behaviors change our genetic expression in return and is a component of inter-generational trauma showing up most clearly in cultures of structured systemic racism.

In this text, almost every case of child sexual abuse (CSA) involves a pattern of multiple betrayals and abandonments of child victims. The cases illustrate a disintegration of protective factors in cultures where the patriarchal domination of women and children is normalized and where bystanders are themselves possessed, groomed, or held in the grip of some blinding, silencing force.

First Episode Psychosis

Breaking from Carrie's story to medically contextualize her psychosis at this point, first episode psychosis simply refers to the time when a person first begins to feel or experience the symptoms of psychosis. This can occur at any time of life, but the first onset is usually in adolescence, with males prone to having an earlier first experience than females (Compton & Broussard, 2009). When the first episode occurs during adolescence, doctors work very hard to ensure that no permanent damage is done to the developing mental and social skills, as adolescence is when social skill building, academic formation, psychological resilience, and self-esteem are learned. As one psychiatrist shared, he has often thought about the destiny of individuals who, once having entered psychosis, never managed to come out of it again.

Early Intervention teams often work with patients for three years, with a provision for extending services if needed. Psychiatric personnel, little known to them, are in a race against the patients' very upbringing (if the patient indeed has sexual abuse in their background), considering the cultural values that have rendered them vulnerable, silenced, and perhaps to return to more of the same cycle.

Carrie's original diagnosis, non-affective psychosis, was defined to include schizophrenia, schizophreniform disorder, brief psychotic disorder, delusional disorder, schizoaffective disorder, and psychotic disorder not otherwise specified. In Carrie's case, the schizotypal personality features of suspicious or paranoid thinking seemed visible in her very pronounced habit of furtive looks and shifty glances.

Compton and Broussard (2009) propose two main models for understanding causes. One is the neurodevelopmental model (involving the developing brain) and the other is the diathesis-stress model (about the relationship between genes and environmental stress). CAP can come out of either. Although Compton and Broussard wrote that "psychosis is a medical condition of the brain, scientists have not figured out exactly what is happening in the brain to cause this illness" (p. 13). More recent research overwhelmingly shows that trauma or adverse childhood experiences affect these changes in the brain.

The three phases of psychosis include the prodromal phase (lasting from weeks to several years), the acute phase, where psychosis manifests in disruptive symptoms and lasts until treatment is sought, and finally, there is the recovery phase, where symptoms hopefully lessen or go away.

In Carrie's case, the positive symptoms of her first visible psychosis (delusion of her body parts floating away, the material world coming apart, and dissociation) cleared up within weeks. However, they returned again and again because, despite institutionalization and a course of medication, the underlying cause of CSA was not factored in. The prodromal signs of anhedonia, apathy, blunted aspect, emotional withdrawal, low energy, slow speech, slow movements, and social isolation were *all* present for most of Carrie's life prior to her breakdown in the city square. Still, this information escaped attending physicians for a variety of reasons.

These signs were also signifiers of the distortion of Carrie's ego-consciousness, which resulted from her abuse. Jung describes ego consciousness as the prerequisite tool for psychological investigation. However, during attempts at psychotherapy, Carrie strenuously avoided taking up any psychic content and holding it in place upon her ego's reflective surface, so to speak. The more Carrie refused to entertain intrusive memories, images, and thoughts, much less to name them, the more a sense of ephemeral transience crept in to "possess" her body and mind.

Reports of Psychosis and Schizophrenia in the Caribbean Diaspora

Reports of high rates of schizophrenia in African Caribbean populations living in urban centers like England show a sixfold risk ratio when compared to white indigenous populations; they are up to 18 times as high for children of African Caribbean immigrants. However, these statistics are often thought to be due to misdiagnosis or to many other etiological factors specific to African Caribbean people living in the United Kingdom.

For example, clinicians understand that positive symptoms of psychosis may be associated with PTSD, but there arises an almost impenetrable cognitive dissonance in applying a diagnosis of psychosis-related PTSD to a child of five or ten because, after all, one thinks, they're surely not old enough to be *post* anything yet! Unfortunately, they may well be, and if this is their case, they may remain unheard, misdiagnosed, and ineffectively treated until the past trauma is finally recognized.

A joint research project between the Universities of Manitoba, Columbia, and Regina examined data on 5,877 people across the United States to determine the rates at which people with PTSD experience psychotic symptoms (Sareen et al., 2005). They found the rate to be approximately 52%. Note that Carrie also experienced every positive symptom listed by these people with PTSD-related psychosis at some stage during the period of sexual abuse by her father. These symptoms include the belief that other people were spying on or following her ("He tracks me, he knows where I am all the time"), seeing something that others could not see (interpreting casual glances or stares from other males as intentions to have forced sex with her), and having unusual feeling inside or outside of her body, such as feeling that she was being touched when no one was really there. Carrie also experienced relentless flashbacks, daydreams, haunted ruminations, and nightmares, believing she could hear what someone else was thinking (expending excessive energy to try to intuit what her abuser was thinking so she could best protect herself from his assaults) and believing that her behaviors and thoughts were being controlled by some power or force (believing the abuser's hypnotic, repeated suggestions that she was born for this, and would forever remain under his spell). Researchers also found evidence that the more PTSD symptoms a person has, the greater the probability of positive psychosis as well. In Carrie's case, CSA could be taken as a predictor for psychosis.

But it was not until Carrie was away from her abuser and in Canada that she loosened the vice grip that she'd kept on her own sanity, praying this new world was a place where she could be caught and saved if she let herself fall. But instead of new beginnings, Carrie was met with the sense of an ending.

Psychosis and Urbanicity

Cities are linked with psychosis for various other reasons as well. Urban centers carry an elevated risk for psychosis, particularly when factors like economic stress, environmental pollutants, and migration or social drift are at play (Heinz et al., 2013; Fett et al., 2019). A range of social factors like social adversity, racism, discrimination, and exclusion are also believed to contribute to mental health challenges (Kirmayer et al., 2010). The full range of factors and the specific ethnic groups they pertain to are largely unknown. If an immigrant to a city is also a refugee, there is an additional probability of distress and trauma carried over from their country of origin. Refugee populations commonly travel to first-world countries, often over perilous routes, to escape poverty, persecution, war, and other forms of oppression or violence. At this moment in history, not only do we witness millions of Syrian and Greek refugees crossing European borders every day, but caravans of undocumented migrants moving stealthily through Latin and South America, Cuba, Haiti, the Dominican Republic, and other places as well. Their common mental health issues include long-lasting conditions of "post-traumatic stress disorder, major depression, generalized anxiety, panic attacks, adjustment disorder, and somatization" (RHTAC, 2011). In this text, I also concern myself with the children of these migratory bodies whose manifestations of trauma do not primarily represent migration alone, neither urbanicity nor other external social factors, but rather describe histories of sex abuse that finally breakthrough in psychosis under the weight of a multiplicity of stressors including geographic displacement.

One of the factors triggering Carrie's breakdown was her sense of non-containment, of de-personalization, of her feeling that her psychic insides were irretrievably emptying into expanses of lakes and highways, never to be gathered up again. Carrie had grown up inside a small house where shutters were perpetually closed to keep out neighbors' prying eyes. Despite the punishing tropical heat, her windows might only be cracked open for a little ventilation as theirs was an architecture of silenced and hidden spaces, and everything in Carrie's perception was constructed upon shuttering. Rooms were small, blinds were drawn, corridors narrow, and verandahs were really too small for much congenial assembling. Streets in her immediate village were barely wide enough for one car to pass without rushing the bushes on either side, and views were kept distant by the thick rain forest irrepressibly pushing in upon her house and yard.

The cultural habit of inhabiting spaces via a series of small, closed rooms does not necessarily have to do with available income for architectural design. Even massive concrete structures are wont to be cut up inside into many small corners. This habit, ostensibly to provide privacy for extended families of numerous relatives, or office buildings where several private meetings are simultaneously conducted, these shuttered spaces work well for molesters and other ill-intended inhabitants who need to cleave to shadows. Patriarchy and mental illness both thrive in such dark and sallow places.

Anima Mundi and the Wild Mind

Depth psychology describes that the landscapes we inhabit shape who we are. They impact our mental health and well-being. Although we live within the rainforest or along coastlines in the Caribbean, a colonized understanding of architecture has barricaded humanity away from the *anima mundi*, denying any form of wildness, whether in the forest or in women and girls. Feminine nature is disallowed its self-agency, and its resources are either exploited for the benefit of man or are spoiled, cut down, and discarded. Contrariwise, indigenous people know our fate to be inseparable from the land we live on and that women have a particular role in nurturing children and the earth. In Celtic tradition, a woman is the guardian of the land and its animals, the bearer of wisdom, and the root of spiritual and moral authority for the tribe. However, in the colonized West, these aspects of the feminine are generally discouraged.

Phenomena like slavery, racism, settler colonialism, and CSA have similar objectives to erase the humanity of the oppressed or, in this context, to erase the humanity of the child.

Jungian poets call for a new understanding of the "wild mind" (Hinton, 2023), in which the entire global ecological crisis is reconceived as a radical rewilding of consciousness itself or a closing of the distance between humankind and nature. Sufi teacher Emmanuel Vaughan-Lee similarly speaks of learning new ways of navigating the unprecedented political and ecological shifts that are upon us, including our connections with nature and with women and girls (Vaughan-Lee, 2023).

Carrie lost her sense of containment and rootedness in the cold, wide expanse of Canadian urbanicity, but she had never felt rooted in her own home at any stage of her life. She had now turned up to begin a new phase of her life and to establish a sense of belonging in a new city, but instead she found that the disembodied specter created by her childhood trauma was now embedded enough to leap forward on its own legs and send her spiraling into a dark, foreboding space.

Back in the evenings of her childhood home, when Carrie silently endured the tortures upon her, she had gathered her split feelings back together like pieces of scrunched cloth and folded herself to sleep, stashing herself in a dark corner with neither ritual, words, nor prayers. Space was nothing that she wanted. There was neither space to think, reflect nor question. She did not ever dream of feeling free but saw herself as a fully surrendered sacrificial lamb. Carrie died every night, there within her shuttered walls, but it was the same death over and again, and she told herself, "I cannot do worse than die".

Jung defines the ego or the body's consciousness of itself as a unique entity, and as such, it is profoundly fearful of the body's death. Child victims, even more so than adult victims, equate rape with death, as one father of a five-year-old female victim told me, "My daughter ruminates without cease. Twenty times a day, she asks me, "Daddy, why did that man try to kill me?""

As Fanon (1952/1968) wrote of himself as a child, following a racist incident with a Caucasian child and its mother, "My body was given back to me sprawled out, distorted, re-colored, clad in mourning" (p. 80).

> (Her) story begins with the body – her body, a place that she was "forced to evacuate when my father invaded and then violated me" … (She) went to sleep with a wary ear – listening for danger, on alert for the … sound of her father's stealthy footsteps in the hall, coming to violate her.
>
> (Bolen, 2014, p. 202)

In Carrie's case, her father had not snatched and manhandled her into forceful sexual encounters such as she had been taught defined rape. Instead, he approached her with a kind of friendliness, sexiness, humility, and insistent pleading. Kenneth Adams described this approach in his book *Silently Seduced* (1991), in which incest predators are not violently abusive strangers who then run away like thieves in the night. Rather, as in the case of Carrie's father, he held her adoringly in his arms and kissed her body just like Carrie saw him do with her mother whenever she stood at their bedroom door watching. She understood this to be the way a man treats his wife, and in her little mind (she was only nine when it started), she believed her father to have married her too, that she was his secret little wife, even more sacred and precious than the first. This is the way that Carrie had been groomed to carry herself. It caused a monstrous sadness to bloom in her, leaving her no room to move, nowhere to look away.

Such careful, strategic grooming includes the purposeful manufacturing of sorrow. If Carrie's ethos could be described in one concept, it would be a dreadful, heavy sorrow, a lingering, despairing wretchedness. Her father worked on damaging the original symbiotic union that his daughter had had with her mother and two sisters, corrupting it forever, a de-civilization of the moral fabric covering the entire family. The mother-child archetype thus rent asunder; the abused child is left without the nourishment, power, or wholeness that would come from a mother-child bond. Instead, a wounded child archetype is born helpless, needy, emotionally crippled, and full of sorrow (Stein, 1973; Myss, 2006). Worse, a victim's relationship with her own instincts is damaged. Such damage obstructs relationships with therapists and the re-unification of the fractured personality in the long term.

> Chagrin was a genuine physical disease. Like a hurt leg or a broken arm … It was not a sudden illness but something that could kill you slowly, Taking a small piece of you every day until one day, it finally takes all of you away.
>
> (Danticat, 2015, p. 23)

Genuine, deep sorrow leaves you torn, confused, hating but loving, guilty, but knowing that you have been wronged. Sorrow confronts you with the betrayal of everything you believed to be sacred while being told that you are nevertheless lucky, that you ought to be grateful, and that this is the way that life must be lived. Sorrow leaves you drained of resistance but somehow, somewhere, still trusting, hopeful, and anxious to appease. One feels guilty for simply being alive. Additionally, being the victim in one situation also sets you up to be victimized by others. Your self-esteem is lowered. Your posture becomes submissive, and any creative endeavors are fraught. You lose the right to say no or to think about no. You are programmed to become a target for the next abusive person who comes along. It is a catastrophic event and one that confronts its victims daily. Being a parent's surrogate partner, as Carrie was, and in cases of mother-son as well as father-daughter incest, a victim is left with feelings of hate, love, and guilt, which together conflate into a rage that is very seldom directly expressed but nevertheless, continues to move and hold sway over the unconscious.

The beginning of the end came one day in high school when Carrie suddenly started screaming. She'd had a good day working on projects she enjoyed with her teachers when the bell rang and the teacher said, "Have a good evening". Carrie's dam suddenly burst. She flung her body backward over her chair and lifted her hips high off the seat, stiff as a board, as though pushing away restraints. Instantly, a community diagnosis of demonic possession was applied, and it sped through the air at the speed of women talking.

Later that day, in the hospital where Carrie had been admitted, no one was more earnest than her father in rushing to her side and petitioning for her release. He was the one to sit by her bedside and spoon-feed her with the "fish braff", he'd made himself while Carrie thought, "This man is a body of water. Any liquid that he puts in me, I have to take". No one saw her hand move with the concealed fork until Carrie had jammed it into his bicep. "Missing his heart", she told me. "I aimed for his heart, but I missed".

He screamed. Her father screamed in a high-pitched, nasal whine, and every nurse coming running thought it must be the girl until they saw her father clutching the instrument that was protruding from his arm.

"Devil!" he snarled, "Satan!" Unexpectedly, he began to pray. Carrie watched him through half-closed eyes and marveled at his ability to call out for Jesus so earnestly and hypnotically that nurses bowed their heads and let him urge the demon in his child to come out in the name of all that was holy.

"Don't touch her!" He told them, arms out-stretched to ward them off. "Don't put a hand! I'm taking her home! We will pray!" Father cried so hard that snot ran from his nose, and he left it to drip. By the next day, "Crazy Carrie" had been discharged to the devoted protection of this father, who now added sermonizing to his hypnotic repertoire. His God-given duty now, he actually articulated, was to pound the devil out of her. Nobody challenged him.

Within the space of 48 hours, Carrie had made three suicide attempts, in addition to the homicidal attack on her father with the fork. Fanon would refer to this as one of the ways in which the colonized being's muscular tension is set free. Gossip spread like wildfire. By the time Carrie's father brought her home from the hospital, everybody had heard of her episode and put their own embellishment on it. "She juk her father in he eye! You hear that? She stab him in he eye!"

Words like strangeness and madness, concepts like being possessed by unseen forces, whether internal or external, and perceptions that sufferers have no powers of logic, no self-control, and are given to violence, cause vulnerable individuals to feel outcast, marginalized, alienized, and without a shred of self-esteem remaining. Quite often, it is this social stigma that hurts the most, not the mental illness itself. Carrie personified all manner of misunderstood terms and conditions and was given a wide berth along with the rest of her family. The village performed its diagnostic test and labeled her mad. Being mortally terrified of madness, they pulled back and left the family to its devices.

> The whole process of being diagnosed with a mental disorder, especially if you have been hospitalized, brings intense feelings of shame … People view you differently, even stigmatize you.
>
> (Mackler & Morrissey, 2010, p. 19)

The natural response in this circumstance is to feel only more shame – and to become silent. But one blessing finally materialized out of this chaos. Carrie's mother finally looked at her squarely and said softly, "Carrie, no school today. We going. Make haste. We going". Mother took Carrie by the right hand and her older sister Melanie by the left, new passports tucked into her bosom, and marched them across the tarmac to an Air Canada jet, only one tote between the three of them. "We going this time", she said. "Come, we going". In the following years, Carrie often wondered how long it had taken her mother to save enough money and gather enough resources to plan an international migration for a whole family in secret. But that day, Carrie held on to her Mum and sprinted for the plane, only to lose herself on a sidewalk upon arriving in the city.

In Canada, where Carrie was indeed caught when she fell and was taken to safety, her diagnostic tests included the Prodromal, Traumatic Life Events Questionnaire (TLEQ), and Basel Screening Instrument for Psychosis (BSIP). All of them asked about background histories of CSA, but no clinician was able to fully relate Carrie's scarcely disclosed history with her current psychological state. Her treatment protocols, therefore, considered her symptoms but not the state of her being. In fact, all of the attributions of the diagnosis had already been on display for years before Carrie's ultimate breakdown, when the rankling bitterness that she carried imploded and was named a psychosis.

When invited, either in individual or group therapy, to share stories of her past, Carrie no longer made any attempt at the truth. She made up and recounted anything she could cling to, speaking like someone with something to hide, her speech marred by inconsistency and shade. The alternative would have been to describe that for seven years, she had been trapped as a sex slave to her father, with both her mother and elder sister apparently knowing and complicit. No school teachers, relatives, or friends noticed her ghostly disintegration and inquired or intervened. During family therapy, neither mother nor sister would confirm Carrie's tales or offer more lucid narratives of their own. All three women of this family fervently denied each other's truths and would not even meet each other in the eye. To Carrie's file was added a notation that there was a heavy genetic loading for psychosis, inclusive of generally low levels of psychological well-being, high levels of anxiety and depression, extremely high levels of interpersonal sensitivity, and co-occurring symptoms of PTSD.

This family constructed a modus operandi of keeping secrets and skeletons in the closet and would not let them out to save their lives. Hence, they felt tainted, as though acceptance outside the confines of the family could only be won by concealment..

In the Canadian institution where Carrie was resident, lovely nature gardens sprawled. But Carrie had never formed an affinity with nature, and she, a Caribbean girl from the edge of a rainforest, professed a terror of bugs and other crawling "beasts". She had also lost an affinity for other women, considering them impotent at best and highly suspicious at worst. As for male doctors and staff, Carrie read them as all-powerful and dangerous. Any friendliness extended by them was taken as immanently sexual in intention, and she amplified her tendency to keep invisible, avoid engagement, and when left no choice, to court appeasement with down-turned, side-shifting glances. To her reputation was added whispers of closeted sexual deviance, and Carrie became socially marginalized even within the margins of residential mental health care. She recognized it and did not mind. This was the comfort zone that she already knew.

Fanon has written of "social therapy" as a practice he initiated with colleagues at Blida, Algeria, a revolutionary move at the time to transform institutionalized psychiatric care. In the context of CAP, a gentle but committed inquiry into this aspect of a patient's background would drive new directions for differential diagnosis and treatment, including the symptoms of post-traumatic sex abuse disorders. However, as I believe Fanon would say, children with CAP still represent "the other" in psychiatric care. "To all intents and purposes (she) represents a system of reference that escapes us … (she) is, in a word, someone that must be treated with consideration because … (her) gaze is unknown, because (she) perhaps has some secret relation … with other people" (Fanon, 2018, p. 380).

During the day, Carrie declined to join other patients in the common spaces, preferring the dim solitude of her room. However, a group of Asians on the grounds outside her window caught Carrie's interest one day. Subsequently, she watched them perform their daily Chi Gong, imitating their movements and painting mandalas with her arms in the air. "Watch it", she often told the nurses who peeked at her as she practiced the forms. "Watch it before I heave this energy at you. I will blast you to pieces with a breath".

The nurses kept their distance. Carrie's eyes were like Medusa's, holding the power to petrify. They had said that about Carrie's eyes all her life; this child had an unknown type of gaze. It was inhospitable.

Social and Environmental Factors

Along with biological factors, such as a history of psychosis in ancestors and family members, which render a person at risk for psychosis or predisposed to the condition of psychosis, there are environmental factors that play a part. Being at genetic risk, or the biological determinants, cannot in themselves alone cause psychosis. The biological factors include not simply genetic material but such diverse criteria as having had a difficult birth or obstetric complication and cannabis use during the gestation of a child. Mainstream medicine has long held out for psychosis being due to chemical imbalances in the brain alone, but more recent research suggests that there must be other social factors that trigger or set the psychosis off (Unger, 2019; Mackenzie, 2021). The list is very long, and it includes urbanicity, separation from parents before the age of 15, bullying, social adversity, and racism, but what we are sure of is that a vulnerability to psychosis generally develops in a person over the years, involving many intersecting conditions before a breakdown actually occurs. Certainly, however, as the case of Bahira in the final chapter will show, there are exceptions to all psychosis rules.

In one small Caribbean island with a population of around 10,000, schizophrenia and bipolar disorder together account for up to 8% of the population of those with poor mental health in the over-20 age category (Pan American Health Organization [PAHO], 2020). In another small island, the most common psychiatric diagnoses are depression, schizophrenia, and drug-induced psychosis (Lamba & Aswani, 2012). Early research into psychosis manifesting in Caribbean people who migrated into the diaspora, like Carrie, indicated that large-scale migration from the Caribbean countries to England in the 1950s to 1960s showed "higher than expected rates of schizophrenia among the African-Caribbean population" (Kiev, 1965; Hemsi, 1967; Bebbington et al., 1981; Cochrane & Bal, 1989). Some researchers claimed that the high incidence of schizophrenia among the African-Caribbean population was due to misdiagnosis by British psychiatrists unfamiliar with Caribbean beliefs and practices (Littlewood & Lepsedge, 1981). Others found that the routine clinical diagnosis of schizophrenia is not a reliable one, though it is not necessarily applied in a racially biased manner (Hickling & Hutchinson, 1999). Maughan (1989) wrote that "African Caribbean children with diagnoses of psychiatric disorders are especially likely to … come from one-parent families, suffered separation from parents, or lived in children's homes or foster homes. However, the etiological significance of these factors is unclear". According to Sharpley et al. (2001), "No simple hypothesis explains these findings". It is, therefore, perhaps more accurate not to describe the illness common among African Caribbeans as classical schizophrenia but to say that this group experiences a type of psychosis whose classification and pathogenesis are unclear up to now. I propose CAP as one explanatory hypothesis, particularly since rates of sexual abuse amongst Caribbean children are given as 47.6% of girls and 31.9% of boys (Jones, 2021).More systematic testing however needs to be carried out.

Psychosis is also now understood to be a common response to severe life disturbances and trauma. Notably, adverse childhood experiences strongly contribute to psychosis (Unger, 2019) or make psychosis much more likely later on. In a recent study, 60–90% of international patients who have psychosis were found to have maltreatment and abuse in their childhoods.

There is no single causal factor for psychosis, but if I could name one predictor based on clinical observation over the years, I would place CSA at the top of the list, even more so than genetic predispositions, as it is true that most people who suffer psychosis have no history of it in their gene pool at all (Mackenzie, 2021). Social defeat is another phenomenon closely associated with psychosis, and victims of incest like Carrie are highly prone.

> Shame is a fundamental emotion. It has been found in all cultures and is recognized by telltale signs: blushing, a lowered head, a sense of unpleasant warmth, downcast eyes, a slack posture, and mental confusion. It is a normal response to feelings of humiliation, disgrace, dishonor, and a sense of inadequacy.
>
> (Mackler & Morrissey, 2010, p. 19)

Postscript

Carrie eventually returned to the island where she was born, unable to make do in the metropolis. She found work in the hospitality industry and lived a simple daily routine, her one remaining social headache being the perpetually irate supervisor at the resort. "Oh God, Carrie! Leave that long, screwed-up face behind you when you come to work! You will frighten the nice tourists. Put on a smile, man, put on a smile!" Carrie would stretch her face to suit, but she remained distracted by the endlessly whispering sound in her ears, like a distant tumbling ocean. Her story continues into the next chapter via elder sister Melanie and younger sister Nightly, whose histories we will now hear.

References

Bolen, J. S. (2014). *Artemis: The Indomitable Spirit in Everywoman*. Conari Press.

Compton, M., & Broussard, B. (2009). *The First Episode of Psychosis: A Guide for Patients and Their Families*. Oxford University Press.

Danticat, E. (2015). *Breath, Eyes, Memory*. Soho Press, Inc.

Fanon, F. (1952/1968). *Black Skin, White Masks*. Penguin Classics.

Fanon, F. (1961). *The Wretched of the Earth*. Grove Press.

Fett, A. J., Lemmers-Jansen, I. L. J., & Krabbendam, L. (2019). Psychosis and urbanicity: A review of the recent literature from epidemiology to neurourbanism. *Current Opinion in Psychiatry*, *32*(3), 232–241. https://doi.org/10.1097/YCO.0000000000000486

Heinz, A., Deserno, L., & Reininghaus, U. (2013). Urbanicity, social adversity and psychosis. *World Psychiatry: Official Journal of the World Psychiatric Association*, *12*(3), 187–197. https://doi.org/10.1002/wps.20056

Hickling, F. W., & Hutchinson, G. (1999). The Roast breadfruit psychosis-disturbed racial identification in African Caribbeans. *Psychiatric Bulletin 23*, 1–3

Kirmayer, L. J., Narasiah, L., Munoz, M., Rashid, M., Ryder, A. G., Guzder, J., Hassan, G., Rousseau, C., & Pottie, K. (2010). Common mental health problems in immigrants and refugees: General approach in primary care. *Canadian Medical Association Journal, 183*(12), E959–E967. https://doi.org/10.1503/cmaj.090292

Lamba, G. S., & Aswani, V. (2012). A case study of mental illness and psychiatric services on the Caribbean Island of Nevis. *International Journal of Mental Health, 41*(4), 24–29. http://www.jstor.org/stable/42003822

Mackler, D., & Morrissey, M. (2010). *A Way Out of Madness: Dealing with Your Family After You've Been Diagnosed with a Psychiatric Disorder*. AuthorHouse.

Myss, C. (2006). *The Language of Archetypes: Discover the Forces that Shape Your Destiny*. Sounds True.

Pan American Health Organization [PAHO]. (2020). *The Burden of Mental Health Disorders in the Caribbean*. https://www.paho.org/sites/default/files/2020-09/MentalHealth-profile-2020%20Grenada_Country_Report_Final.pdf

Romme, M., & Escher, S. (Eds.). (2013). *Psychosis as a Personal Crisis: An Experience-Based Approach*. Routledge.

Sareen, J., Cox, B. J., Goodwin, R. D., & Asmundson, J. G. (2005). Co-occurrence of post-traumatic stress disorder with positive psychotic symptoms in a nationally representative sample. *Journal of Traumatic Stress, 18*(4), 313–322. https://doi.org/10.1002/jts.20040

Sharpley, M., Hutchinson, G., Murray, R. M., & McKenzie, K. (2001). Understanding the excess of psychosis among the African-Caribbean population in England. *British Journal of Psychiatry, 178*(S40), s60–s68. https://doi.org/10.1192/bjp.178.40.s60

Unger, R. (2019). *Introducing the Evidence that Trauma Can Cause Psychosis* [Video]. YouTube. https://www.youtube.com/watch?v=x4tCPFFm9VE

Chapter 2

Melanie

Impact on Families

Carrie's older sister, Melanie, was the first family member to voluntarily seek psychotherapy, and she was in her late 50s at the time. Most female victims of child sexual abuse (CSA) make their first report at an average age of 52, regardless of how young they were at the onset. Melanie is considered a victim because although she was never directly abused or mistreated herself, she had witnessed it all from the start.

> The tension of a mysterious danger is even more unbearable than danger itself. People … want security. They even prefer war to the insecure expectation of a war with its threat of enemy surprise.
>
> (Joost Meerloo)

"I just can't take it again". Melanie, age 58, wept dry, scratchy tears. It was as though the event was unfolding before her eyes at that very time. "When is it going to stop? Night after night after night, I just hid in the closet, watching my sister flopping around like a fish in a pail, begging for her life. Her voice is still ringing in my ears. What that man was doing to her, how could she take it? I just sat there and prayed. I peed myself. When was it going to stop?" Melanie drew a deep, shuddering breath. "I feel as though mice are nibbling away at the edges of my mind. Cockroaches are fluttering in my brain. I'm getting mad".

Melanie was experiencing a crushing guilt, but not because she'd been an immobile bystander. Instead, she felt that remaining silent *caused* her sister's torments. Melanie was carrying *perpetrator* guilt and self-loathing because of it.

After the Holocaust, we learned the term "Survivor Guilt" with all of its implications, and after the COVID-19 pandemic, we named a new diagnosis "Prolonged Grief Disorder". We have yet to name the disorders manifesting in members of families who witness and remain silenced around incest in their homes. However, a closer study of this phenomenon would help us understand the prevalence of disorders that accompany bystander complicity in families where incest is practiced.

Long after Melanie's mother took herself and Carrie and fled their abusive home, Melanie continued to be haunted by guilt. Worse, along with guilt, she wrestled to

DOI: 10.4324/9781003223603-4

understand why she simultaneously felt jealous of Carrie, the one their father had selected to favor, groom, and torture. Melanie felt that father and sister shared a bond she would never know and the dark complexity of these feelings drove her mad. Over the years, even as she married and bore a child of her own ("Oh no, not a daughter!"), Melanie continued slipping into a shadowy, brooding realm of resentment and non-being. Complexes, according to Jung, are precisely these highly charged emotional knots that burrow into the unconscious and nestle there.

The Father Complex

In Melanie's Father Complex, regarding the specific wound of a "monstrous father", the ego experiences itself as eternally young, small, and without agency; a collapsed child or eternal *puella*, as Jung might say. The position is so painful to bear that the child unconsciously moves to inhabit the father's negative position and then begins to move through the world abusing people in the way that her father did. Melanie did not become sexually abusive to anyone, but as she grew into adulthood, she became eviscerating, cruel, and even menacing to colleagues and friends. In fact, Melanie switched between the two polarities, on the one hand being the collapsed and frightened child victim, and on the other hand, triggered by an impetus that only she could see, she visited versions of the same demeaning and brutal traits with which she and her sister had been raised. Her chronically poor relationship patterns left Melanie isolated, lonely, and consequently frustrated and angry. She ran between chasing friends for their companionship in a fawning manner and viciously lashing out at them, or speaking badly about them, when she felt slighted or rejected. Worse, she was unable to see her own shadow at play. She was particularly vicious with other women, and as her own daughter grew, Melanie struck and swore at her as the toxic trajectory wore on unabated. As several psychologists have written, mothers who have experienced sexual abuse have great difficulty in the parental role and lower levels of parental efficiency..

During Melanie's sleepless nights, when she got out of bed and paced the corridors, her husband saw her talking to herself in the same tone her father had. Melanie's self-talk was critical, crushing, and derisive. When she finally committed herself to therapy, she would be called upon to bring her destructive behaviors into conscious awareness and to recognize that she had become what she most hated. However, as is normal in cases like these, Melanie hid behind her collapsed child complex (notice the conflation of several elements in the complex). She turned viciously against the therapist's attempts to have her face her own shadow when she suggested that Melanie was, in fact, "possessed" by her father's energy and was re-enacting his destruction in her world as well.

In cases like Melanie's, where early child incest is at the root of a psychotic breakdown later in life, if the visible symptoms of psychosis are treated alone, without attention to the psychological complexes that always accompany child abuse, such as the father wound, the mother wound, or both, the victim could never conceivably achieve fulsome healing.

The Mother Wound

It is not usual to suffer from both father and mother wounds, but in cases of incest by one parent where the other parent fails to intervene, both wounds may manifest simultaneously. A woman with a mother wound, like Melanie, suffers from issues of control and perfectionism. She selects a man with a strong feminine side to experience the sweetness and unconditional love she did not receive from her mother and to compensate for the selective blindness and muteness experienced in her family, Melanie became hyper-vigilant, loud, intrusive, and interfering. Furthermore, lest she leave any dark corners un-swept, she randomly swung her broom about like nunchaku accusing everyone of everything. Most confusing to anyone in her purview was her capacity to collapse in the middle of fully aggressive actions, leaving people bewildered and running after her to offer comfort after she had just savaged them. Lately, however, people were increasingly walking away, leaving her in a puddle. Only David always remained, with his quiet feminine energy.

To complicate the complex further, Melanie would turn around and berate David for being too soft and for not wearing the pants in the family. "I have to do everything around here" she would sob. "I have to see everything, hear everything, run to fix everything. You need to pull your pants up!" David's gentle response, invariably, was, "Baby, there is nothing to see, hear or fix in this house. Try to calm down". And their daughter, watching from the doorway with a severe mother wound of her own, would mutter, "What a cunt".

A mother wound may also be defined as a cultural trauma created by a patriarchal society that is oppressive or violent toward women. This is clearly applicable to all of the women in this family, spanning three generations, because of the behavior of the one male predator among them, along with society's many silencing and normalizing mechanisms along the way. But healing from this involves unraveling the frustration, rage, *and* love that come wrapped up in each individual constellation, including the development of the deeply embedded personality disorders that frequently ensue.

If a psychotic breakdown occurs, as in the dramatic public case of Carrie or the private, internal combustion of Melanie, only a Depth Psychological approach, in combination with medical treatments, has a chance of getting to the root.

The Night Mutterer: Happiness Denied

Under the comfort of darkness, when Melanie believed her household to have surrendered to their peaceful dreams, she let go of all pretenses of truth, talking to herself in words that would never see daylight.

When someone comes home alone at night or is suddenly awakened by a loud noise and calls out, "Who's there?" this is not because an answer is expected but because the sound of one's own voice provides a level of comfort and grounding that no one else's can. Melanie spoke to herself in the darkness, pacing up and down, venting to the many currents running through her brain, memory, and skin.

She fantasized, made up stories, devised lies she knew were lies, and spun them into tales she told herself, making crochet out of her eclipsed realities. Routinely, she set up half the night, spitting and muttering at the shadows. She lurched from one narrative to the other, then doubled back to respond to a point she'd made several hours before. Her speech pattern was like a diamond kite in the Easter breeze, loosening out and upwards with bird's flight speed, then plunging from one side to the other in the currents without tail-rudder or keel. None but the wind could ever keep up with Melanie in her nighttime rants, and she needed no further accompaniment than that.

Melanie's inner child perpetually returned to where it had first felt stuck: a closeted, darkened space within which she had "smalled up" herself, stifled and suffocating but unable to resist peeking. These days, as she paced the midnight corridor of her adult home, she spoke in the way she would have then if she could have. In her hallway was a long, narrow Anatolian rug heavily invested with the symbols and visual narratives of a mystical life. These are the symbols that Melanie petitioned and quarreled with when she assumed the household was fast asleep in their beds.

Symbolism and Spiritualistic Experiences

At the dawn of the 20th century, visual and literary artists joined psychologists in exploring symbolisms and other art forms alongside dreams, fantasies, and visions to find expanded insights into the actualities of inner experience. Carl Jung's Liber Novus, or the Red Book (published in 2009), speaks to his exploration of the psychogenesis of spiritualistic phenomena or the psychological origins of states of psychic possession. An early discovery was that regardless of whether the alleged spiritualistic experiences were valid, such experiences enabled far-reaching insights into the constitution of the subliminal, and hence into human psychology as a whole" (Jung & Shamsasani, 2009, p.195). Jung's research, while situated at the Burghölzli, which included automatic writing, trance speech, and his work as a fine artist, helped concretize his understanding of schizophrenia as "an intelligibility of delusion formations" (CW 3). He wrote, "If we feel our way into the human secrets of the sick person, the madness also reveals its system, and we recognize in the mental illness merely an exceptional reaction to emotional problems which are not strange to us" (CW 3, 339). When Jung left employment as a psychiatrist at Burghölzli to further his personal research, he incorporated myth, religion, and folklore in his psychoanalytical work.

Melanie's midnight rants, in which she deliberately dissociated from reality to correspond with the symbols on the carpet, may be described as imagistic or thinking in pictorial form. In Jung's language, she engaged herself in active imagination and held inner dialogues. Whether she painted her mandalas and visions as Jung had, externalizing the contents of his unconscious, or wandered through labyrinths of symbols made by others as in her slow, incessant pacing of the Persian rug, Melanie's process was *both* a letting go and a holding on. She was letting go of her inherited reality as having any legitimate life-giving capacity for her and reaching out for other worlds that might offer a new framework.

If anyone other than a depth psychologist (or artist, or indigenous person) had witnessed these flights of fantasy of Melanie's, they would certainly have labeled her psychotic or demon-possessed.

From his corner, unseen, as her husband listened to the ravings, he felt an overwhelming burden of sadness overtake him, a sadness that was still trickling down from the deliberate cultivation of it that Melanie and Carrie's father initiated when he began to corrupt their lives. As Brewster (2020) wrote, even two generations of trauma will send that trauma down a line of descendants for many more generations to come.

If psychosis means a complete break with reality, David told himself, my wife schedules herself an episode once daily. All else around them reflected the prestige of David's position as chief executive officer (CEO) of an accountancy firm. He was a tall, lean, raw-boned man with a bald pate, a carefully groomed long red beard, and a calm, conscientious demeanor. Melanie had been attracted to him for his controlled, stoic manner. Where his first wife had abandoned him because he was "emotionally unavailable", this was the quality that Melanie desired most. Had he been a eunuch, she would have loved it all the more. This relates to Jung's Repetition Compulsion, in which someone with an emotionally distant or abusive parent or caregiver goes on to have adult relationships with people who are distant, too. Repetition compulsion is discussed in more detail in the chapter on The Boy.

Melanie and David met at university, where they first talked for hours over chocolate lattes. They later shared glasses of red wine at the side of their professor's fire, where he ran graduate seminars from the comfort of his Rosedale home.

David played the archetypal role of Nurturer, especially to his wife and their daughter. As far back as he could remember, he was an empath, sensitive to the feelings of others, including his parents and siblings, as well as his wife and child. Although the relationship dynamic between himself and Melanie begs for much further expansion, it suffices to say here that David had chosen to partner with someone distinctly not his emotional or physical equal, as his early-assigned relationship role was that of caretaker. Regarding her physicality, Melanie was blessed with a classical, somewhat aloof beauty, but medical ailments beset her. The umbrella diagnosis was fibromyalgia, but a host of other disorders ebbed and flowed in that wake. As Gabor Maté has said,, women contract over 80% of all known autoimmune diseases, which tend to befall people who are compulsively concerned with suppressing healthy anger and maintaining a sense of duty and responsibility to others at their own expense. In Melanie's case, her failure to act responsibly toward her younger sister's abuse kept her locked in an obsessive compulsion to care for everyone else and to be seen, acknowledged, and admired for that care. The rage she carried against her parents, and herself caught her in a swell of such complex resentments that she could not make head or tail of it all.

Anger is a boundary defense mechanism, Maté suggests, meaning that expressing anger healthily is good for the neurological system and its physiological response. If you repress your emotions, you simultaneously repress your immune system, which is undermined as far as not recognizing malignancy when it encounters it. Hence, Melanie was sick all the time.

David so conscientiously attended all of these complications that if disrupted from his role at all, he could fairly easily spiral into his own mental health crisis as he had done before meeting Melanie. His fastidious control of the energies and behaviors in his home was equally for his own salvation as for those in his care. As such, David never truly sought to help heal Melanie, or he feared he would have no meaningful role in her life, but certainly, he did try to keep her hidden from the harm of others. "Never mind what everybody says about you, baby", he often told her, "I am always here for you. Never forget that. Till death do us part". The codependent relationship suited them both quite well.

David was as meticulous with his personal routine as he was with his customers' finances, and all around him were the accouterments of his success. If any of the gods could be thought to inhabit this space, David thought, considering his walls ranged with books covering topics from Greek antiquity through modern African Sci-Fi, it would be Apollo, master of harmony and order. However, instead, here we had Melinoë herself, the aptly named bringer of nightmares and madness. Years later, to his shock, Melanie told him she had known he was watching her pacing the corridor all along. "Of course, I saw you!" She snapped at him bitterly. "You over-flowed the doorway!".

We all have the potential for our psyches to break with reality when traumatized. Unconscious contents flood our egos to the point where the ego can no longer navigate the unrestrained chaos in our minds, and cracks in our armor appear. But it is often the awareness and fear of the condition rather than the condition itself that cripples victims, as in the case of Melanie. She was entirely aware of her issues, hence the careful containment of them during the nighttime hours in her closet, rather, her corridor. If Melanie were asked to name her single most dominant emotion, she would call it panic.

Depth Psychology and the Mythical Tradition

It is important to note that gods and goddesses are not referenced by any mythologists or scholars as though they are real existing entities. Instead, they are myths that are expressive of humankind's collective unconscious, which is why cultures from opposite ends of the earth may share myths and legends that are strikingly similar. Whether speaking of Zeus from Greek mythology, Eshu from the Yoruba and Dogon peoples of Africa, Quetzalcoatl of the Aztec civilization, or Raven, one of the celestial beings of Canada's Haida myths, the core ideas expressed in these archetypes reflect commonly held human thinking. As one Canadian chief explains:

> When you have learned all that language can convey, there are still a thousand images, suggestions, and associations recurring to the Indian.
>
> (Clark, 1960, p. xii)

Storytelling and mythology are thus vital parts of the depth psychology tradition, together with dreams being the *Via Regia* or royal road to the unconscious, as Jung has said. In my work as a psychologist, along with drawing from neurobiological understandings of how trauma affects the brain and body; how child abuse psychosis originates and proceeds, and how cognitions and behaviors may twist, shatter, and come back together again, I find deep relevance and richness in the wisdom of cultural myths whose tellers have recorded concepts describing the human condition from the very dawn of time.

David had suspected his wife even more deranged than she let on, but during the daylight, she was a past master at faking it. Though she dropped out of law school once they married, she managed their mortgages, the household, and the social calendar with impressive conscientiousness and ease. However, she was much less capable of human relationships, having alienated almost all her friends by this time. She had stopped having intimate relations with David the moment their one child was conceived ("Sex is an evil thing", she told him in no uncertain terms). These days, instead of aging like fine wine, Melanie was maturing into dysfunction, and she courted her own possession by a dark aspect of the feminine divine.

The Dark Feminine

Melinoë is the name of a lesser-known goddess. In my work with child victims of chronic incestuous abuse, particularly where the abuse begins at a very early age and is either of an overt or covert nature, Melinoe manifests as a powerful and helpful archetypal energy.

The term archetype is a "hypothetical construct used to account for the similarity in the images that cluster around typically human themes and situations, whether cross-culturally, in the dreams of modern people, in children's drawings, or the delusions of psychotics" (Brooks, 2015, p. 17). Common archetypal figures are the mother, the hero, the divine child, the wise older woman, and so on. The mythic gods and goddesses are also archetypes. In depth psychology, the archetypes serve as potentialities of the self and are sources of tremendously powerful psychic energy. Note that not all archetypes are "nice", but they are all exceedingly powerful.

Melinoë is a Chthonic goddess. Chthonic is derived from the Greek word *khthon*, meaning earth or soil. A Chthonic god or goddess is, therefore, one who dwells within or beneath the earth. They are smoldering gods that inhabit deep, dark places, hidden from mortal eyes and influences. Melinoë is first mentioned in the Orphic Hymns of the 2nd or 3rd century A.D. Athanassakis and Wolkow (2013) and is represented as a bringer of nightmares and madness. Described as half black and half white (notice the reference to melanin), Melinoe is the daughter of Zeus and his own daughter Persephone (see the reference to incest), who is the goddess of death.

The Orphic hymns are a collection of 87 short religious poems addressed to various deities and belong to a canon of Orphic literature that centers around the mythical hero, Orpheus, a poet and musician. (We will see Orpheus show up again as the story of Yara unfolds.) As Orphism developed into an ancient mystery school where Greek scholars like Plato and Socrates pondered theories of the soul, the word psyche came into being, the Greek word for soul. The original meaning and function of the term psyche-logos, or psychology, thus meant a study of the soul.

Another new term, *metempsychosis*, came into being in the teaching of Pythagoras, meaning the immortality or reincarnation of the human soul or the transmigration of the human soul at death. This term did not come into active usage until the late 16th century, from the Greek word *metempsukhosis*, broken down into meta – expressing change + en – in + psukhe – soul. Understanding this ancient concept of psychosis as a release of the soul from the body allows me to take it as an apt description of the psychotic split or break that Carrie repeatedly experienced under the horror-stricken gaze of her sister Melanie, where she "flopped around like a fish in a pail begging for her life". This indicates that child abuse psychosis may be seen as something not unnatural to either biology or spirit but as an expected result of immanent psychic death, real or perceived. As Carrie articulated, "I die every night. I cannot do worse than this".

In the case of Melanie, she never contemplated death. Rather, she reached deep down into her unique soul, into her personal and collective unconscious, and tapped into a feminine archetypal energy that is ferocious, not appeasing; that slays, not acquiesces; that looks and sounds like what Westerners may name demonic possession (or psychosis), and thus they shame, ridicule and medicate the condition.

Melanie eventually found a psychotherapist with the safe, non-judgmental space that she had needed all her life, and her story finally came out, but the disclosure of incest (Melanie's being covert; her sister Carrie's being overt) did not come out front and center, but from deep within a complex assortment of symptoms, signs and manifestations of post-traumatic distress that had remained submerged even during the group therapy processes in Carrie's Canadian institution. They finally burst out in individual psychotherapy, when at least three generations of the women in this family had been almost destroyed. As Hollis wrote, "Unconsciousness of one's trauma causes one to wound oneself repeatedly", along with others (Hollis, 1996, p. 79).

A third sister existed, the youngest child about whom very little was ever told except that her name was Nightly. She was spirited away from the home as an infant by a maternal aunt who descended on the household one day, bringing hell and damnation. Carrie and Melanie remember a knock-down, drag-out fight between Mother and Auntie. Words like "Not again! Not this one too!" were flung, and by the end of an extensive cursing session, Auntie burst into the girls' shared room, grabbed Nightly up, and sailed off with her in arms, colorful baubles bouncing up and down on her braids as they went. "Try to stop me!" Auntie screamed as mother flung herself at her sister, dragging at the legs of her youngest baby girl. "Mummy dragged off one of Nightly's shoes", Melanie told me. "God knows that one little pink shoe is probably in the bush there still". But Auntie and infant disappeared down the road, not to be seen or heard from again for many years.

More than a decade passed before the three sisters met again. Old suspicions and fears that were previously buried boiled up to the surface and erupted. There began an extremely painful sojourn of reconnection, but Nightly found herself ganged up on and stigmatized by the older two, and she had clarity enough to recognize it. It was not a stigma against the mental illness that seemed to characterize all the women in this family, but a stigma against mental *health*. The child *had* overcome her trauma; that was her sin. She was too free, too confident, too unbothered. It made the older two and their mother look bad, and they collectively resented it. In whatever nuanced and underhanded ways they could, they gas-lighted, isolated, and punished her for this freedom.

Postscript

This family of four women was first introduced to individual psychotherapy by Melanie in her late 50s. Mother, Melanie, Carrie, and Nightly came to sessions independently during this time in Toronto and overseas. The Aunt who had taken Nightly away also dipped in from time to time. Carrie eventually returned to the land of her birth, managing a job and a home. Though she remained fearful of people in general and lived as any anti-social, paranoid individual might, the fact that she could open the windows of her house to let in light and air, and sit on her verandah in the evenings to enjoy a little breeze marks significant progress.

Melanie remains in the watchful care of her husband. Still, she attends therapy with a new focus on healing the relationship with her estranged daughter, who still elects to stay in her boarding school even over the holidays, referring to her mother as a "vicious, unhealed, tyrannical witch". It would become clear, over the years, that Melanie suffered more deeply from her mother's wound than her father's, and the links between that betrayal and her behavior with her own child were very challenging to face.

Nightly, the youngest sister, pops in now and then as she travels internationally for work and has achieved all of the objectives, she has set for herself thus far. Still, she remains haunted by a cloying, impenetrable sorrow that washes over her out of the blue sometimes.

Mother has not been able to rid herself of her guilt and regret. She drinks heavily and enjoys the therapy of pharmaceuticals but occasionally craves the release of a full nervous breakdown and schedules a therapist to witness and contain her.

As for the father, the single causal factor of all of this wretchedness, he simply has passed into absolute irrelevance; no one thinks of him or calls his name.

References

Athanassakis, A., & Wolkow, B. (2013). *The Orphic Hymns*. John Hopkins University Press.
Brewster, F. (2020). *The Racial Complex: A Jungian Perspective in Culture and Race*. Routledge.

Brooks, J. (2015). *Learning from the Lifeworld*. The British Psychological Society. https://www.bps.org.uk/psychologist/learning-lifeworld

Clark, E. (1960). *Indian Legends of Canada*. McClelland and Stewart.

Hollis, J. (1936). *Under Saturn's Shadow: The Wounding and Healing of Men*. Inner City Books.

Jung, C. G., & Shamdasani, S. (Ed.). (2009). *The red book: Liber novus* (M. Kyburz & J. Peck, Trans.). W W Norton & Co.

Chapter 3

Bystander Mobilization

Bystander Mobilization in Context

In Latin America and the Caribbean (LAC), as in many parts of the world, violence against women and children has become normalized.

Vulnerable populations report that when neighbors witness harm occurring, they often choose not to take decisive, helpful action for a multiplicity of reasons. While victims of chronic abuse report that "somebody always knew," whole segments of a village may remain silenced, immobilized, and thereby complicit in the violence. Considering community mobilization as a social theory, or even as a social justice movement, has the potential to explain why that is, particularly in cultures with a history of imperialism, colonialism, and strong patriarchal processes that typically hold obedience and loyalty as core values. Social constructionist theory, the theory of planned behavior, and psychoanalytic transformative learning are also theoretical frameworks that help navigate this puzzling domain and answer why family members remain frozen and collapsed while grievous bodily harm is perpetrated on others, and how do we mobilize populations of bystanders to take action to protect families and neighbors from violence, thereby improving health outcomes and issues for victims in the LAC region and the wider world.

My introduction to the concept of the apathetic bystander initially came through readings of the Jewish Holocaust many years ago. I was particularly moved by Ellie Wiesel's Nobel Prize acceptance speech on Europe's indifference to the sufferings of the Jews, in which he compared blame for the perpetrators of the Holocaust to blame for the bystanders, which Wiesel believed to be of equivalent evil. Most of the literature I consumed was emotionally fraught, counting those who wrote of the profound and ubiquitous hatred that they believed bystanders must feel for those they silently watched get tortured and killed, and those who later called for a scientific inquiry into the emotional ties that bind victims to perpetrators. Bourke, for example, pulled from psychoanalytic theories to show how attachment plays a crucial role in whether bystanders (or victims) may mobilize to help themselves and each other. On the opposite end of the spectrum, more recent research coming out of America and mainly focused on sexual abuse on American college campuses presents evidence that bystanders do intervene

DOI: 10.4324/9781003223603-5

all the time. However, the interventions are not always successful (Moschella & Banyard, 2020) as it was found that success depends largely upon interpersonal relationships.

The complexity of interpersonal dynamics regarding bystander behavior was also explored by Guiora (2017), who, like myself, considers both deeply personal and theoretical perspectives on victims' rights. Guiora led with ethnographic material from his parents and grandparents, who were survivors of the Holocaust and pushed to make non-intervention a crime and punishable by law. Guiora (2020) then took an unflinching look at institutional enablers of sexual violence in America, revealing how bystander behavior is not accidental but deliberately and strategically constructed for the benefit of perpetrators. The title of his book itself tells a full tale: *Armies of Enablers: Survivor Stories in Complicity and Betrayal in Sexual Assault* (2020).

Guiora's point of view gave me pause and is painful to contemplate, as child sexual abuse (CSA) is similarly described as a normalized social construct in accordance with the attitudes and behaviors that allow patriarchal systems of power, control, and violence to flourish unchallenged. Guiora answered the hard question of whether law and morality should compel action against the consequences of hatred (Friedman, 2020). Though heart-wrenching in their raw exposure of deeply troubling facts, Guiora's texts (2017/2020) presented a clear legal route for enforcing bystander mobilization.

Two central perspectives emerge as crucial to understanding how to break intrafamilial silence, such as in Carrie and Melanie's childhood home. First is the overwhelming and enduring rage that victims of violence feel against those who stand by indifferently and allow harm to happen to them (those often being siblings, nonoffending parents, and/or other family members), and second is the evidence that many bystanders, at home or in the community, would act much more decisively to help potential victims if only they knew what actions to take safely, given the nuanced complexities of relationships within various inter-personal dynamics and social contexts.

One of these nuanced complexities in the realm of academia is that the term "bystander mobilization" seems to have slipped away from public discourse and to a large extent has been replaced by terms like "pro-social behavior" (Atienzo et al., 2018; Chaney, 2020; Jones, 2021; Hulley et al., 2022) and "positive deviancy" (Zuckerhut, 2018; Polsky, 2022). This new language speaks to the same focus, though using a different lens. In my opinion, the new terms lack urgency and do not quite touch the heart of the conflict. They may be more tolerable in terms of abstract concepts, but "bystander mobilization" seems more of a compelling call to action. The central issue remains how to arrest normalized violence against vulnerable individuals and groups and create a movement that mobilizes or deviates bystanders away from apathetic observation and toward pro-social behaviors. This movement would build upon the primary prevention movement in CSA, which asserts that when people have accurate knowledge about CSA, they will be better able to identify it and intervene to stop it.

Finding the mental, intellectual, emotional, and financial resources necessary to take on these fraught and deeply complex psychosocial constructs is extremely challenging when the population is already strained with other pressing demands. In the LAC, crime levels are extraordinarily high, a fact that nationals have grappled with for decades if not hundreds of years. One in four citizens claim fear of violence as their major social concern above unemployment or the state of the economy (Jitman & Machin, 2015; Pérez & Rasch, 2020). The annual rate of homicide is more than three times the world's average, and taking America as an example of the world average, in 2015, 36% of American women experienced intimate partner violence at some point in their lifetime, and 21% of them have experienced an attempted or completed rape (Decker et al., 2018). Additionally, recent statistics claim that 40 of the 50 most dangerous cities in the world are in the LAC (Statista, 2022).

This makes the region uniquely paradoxical since it is at once a busy tourist destination and simultaneously extremely dangerous in some areas. High crime levels lead to costly behavioral responses within the general population, including decreased natural pro-social tendencies and onlooker apathy (Bar-On, 2001; Blazquez & Le Cour Grandmaison, 2021). Furthermore, Flecha (2021) described second-order sexual harassment (SOSH) as a key factor in the construction of social silencing. SOSH refers to harassment of those who stand with victims of violence or violence to the silence-breakers. On a much wider sphere, the wars of cancellation, banning, blocking, and boycotting that have broken out on social media in the last months of 2023 in response to Israel's behavior in Palestine illustrates the systemic role that second-order harassment can play on a world stage, having potential for both harm and good.

In the LAC, over 600 years of slavery and imperialism by the British, French, Spanish, and Portuguese have left a legacy of dominance and oppression, and patriarchal control has become normalized in all of the diverse populations (Lacey et al., 2019). McBride et al. (2022) wrote about the theory of planned behavior as "the behavioral process of planning and preparing to commit an act of terrorism or targeted violence often culminating in the perpetration of such acts" (McBride et al., 2022, p. 25). I argue that this scholarship may be broadened to include child abuse, particularly in instances of chronic and catastrophic incest-related violence carried out on children over the years as planned acts of terror. According to START (The National Consortium for the Study of Terrorism and Responses to Terrorism, 2019), the theory of planned behavior explains how groups or isolated individuals may be mobilized toward acts of violence or trained away from them. Again, I am sure that this relates to child abuse as it does to war. We have copious amounts of literature on victims, victim mentality, and victim healing, but we have comparatively none on perpetrators or on the systems that allow them to plan and execute rapes that remain silenced and normalized over the years. We know how many victims exist in various demographics, say one in three girls in America prior to the age of 18 and one in five in England and Wales, but how many perpetrators exist within any one village, community, or space? The theory of planned behavior certainly needs to be applied here, including to researchers who only investigate in one direction.

My personal experience with constructed, strategic silence came when I was ten years old, and my girl friend and I ran through a densely treed avenue between her home and mine. We played our usual game as we ran: ten hops, ten skips, ten scissors' switches, and so on, taking turns to call out each next series. These were the years of gleeful exuberance, and our laughter rang out as we skipped along. Then, a young man emerged from the bushes ahead. He was calm, slow, and methodical as he walked toward us, calling out recriminations. All I remember of the monologue is that it was directed toward my friend's father. This high court judge had recently delivered a verdict that this man evidently found unfair. Frozen in our tracks, we watched him walk up and slap my friend so hard in the face that she somersaulted backward. I, as a bystander, could do nothing. I was frozen by the first act of violence I had ever seen, and as I struggled to make sense of *why* it had happened, I didn't move. Then, the young man turned his calm eyes upon me. "You are the same," he said. The slap to my face flung me across the road, and as I landed, I saw neighbors coming out and looking on but doing nothing. I, as a victim, could only think of getting away fast. My friend was already on the move, and I followed her, unbelievably resuming the hop, skip, and jump game just where we had left off, minus exuberance.

Once home, I immediately told one of my older brothers and witnessed all hell unleash. Up on his feet and running for my father in the blink of an eye, they both emerged with weapons, wild eyes, and hell to pay. My mother ran behind, calling to them and Jesus with equal urgency, warning of repercussions and ongoing hell to pay. They all turned toward me now, demanding a description of the man and his precise location.

Riddled with confusion, de-personalized and petrified of this brand-new chaos, my adolescent impulse to self-assertion arose, and in so doing, it affirmed the power with which the world was confronting me. My family perceived their collective identity to be threatened, and they were going to take power back without any concern for me, the victim. These fiercely protective, loving men in my family chose to behave in a vengeful, ruthless, imperialistic, and selfish manner, or so I saw it. To protect them in return, I chose to give the wrong description of the man, along with an imprecise location. Thus, I reclaimed my self-determination in the only way I knew how; I perpetrated silence, misinformation, and lies.

Although my girlfriend and I have never spoken of the incident, it still haunts me. My understanding of bystander mobilization has been constructed with a concrete, insider perspective of the intensely complex dynamic between victim, perpetrator, and people looking on. From this standpoint, I have witnessed myself construct an understanding of families and society. I cannot but stand with psychoanalytic scholarship, which calls for a deeper understanding of this interpersonal problem before bystanders can successfully be engaged or mobilized. Additionally, my experience has informed my preference for the term "bystander mobilization" over "prosocial behavior" (Blazquez & Le Cour Grandmaison, 2021) since, in my mind, it *was* a pro-social choice to thwart my family's intentions to seek vengeance on my behalf.

Bystander mobilization has powerful implications for interrupting an oppressive paradigm and pointing the way to the conscientization that Freire (1970) articulated over 50 years ago, which remains the backbone of our scholarship in adult education today. Similarly to Friere, the social constructionist paradigm sees problems as created rather than objectively existing (Evans, 2000), therefore urging a way to extract, mobilize or elicit the good that exists in all individuals.

Since significant personality change occurs through the exploration of various parts of the psyche and through integrating the ego with other personality elements and societal factors to achieve wholeness, this methodological approach is tailor-made for population impact in places like the global south. However, as psychoanalytic transformative learning only sometimes provides the systematic scaffolding necessary for effecting large-scale social transformation within the field of adult education within prescribed timelines, working with methodologies to effect bystander mobilization requires the full scope of a multi-disciplinary framework.

In 1996, bystanders were defined in relation to their role in the abuse of victims. That is, where they were neither victim nor perpetrator, they were counted as onlookers who, by remaining on the sidelines became complicit with the abuser (Salmivalli et al., 1996). In 1998, Oleweus made the point that such situations always involved an imbalance of power, in which victims of the power dynamic could not easily defend themselves; thus, the abuse (including bystander immobility) was repeated over time. This early literature is particularly relevant as it considers victims of incest in which the grooming, complicity, and normalization of abuse generally continue repeatedly over time – even up to 15 or 21 years of age (of the victim). By 2015, the theory of bystander intervention had been developed to focus succinctly on mobilizing peers to defend victims in various different scenarios and formats. For example, the term bystander passivity was used to describe situations of racist violence, and Price (2014) coined the term "hybrid bystander" to include cyber bullies as well.

Regarding more general issues of violence against vulnerable people, Nelson et al. (2011) described the role of "group identity" in the enablement of racist violence in terms of a strong religious emphasis on keeping families united and strong in the face of numerous social threats, both self-inflicted and external. We have a high rate of teenage pregnancies in which the teenagers are expelled from school (rather, shamed into not returning), and barriers are constructed to frustrate the completion of their education. Additionally, it is normal to find single mothers of numerous children (up to nine or more) from multiple fathers, none of whom are present or contributing, and there is escalating youth crime with children as young as nine already in conflict with the law and in juvenile detention. Though not mentioned by Nelson et al., I equate their "group identity" concept to bystander complicity in sexual abuse crimes, where the punishment of offenders would result in the tangible disruption of their families (perpetrators sentenced to jail and/or victims removed to foster care), such disruption being actively condemned by many church and state communities, and by neighbors, not to mention the perpetrators themselves.

Oxhorn (1999) brought forward a salient point regarding the "multifaceted marginalization of substantial segments of the populations" (p. 129). In reference to the fact that most statistics on violence are collected from those who actually report incidences, that is, people who are already disenfranchised in society, Oxhorn asks, "What is the role of the popular sectors or lower classes?" (Oxhorn, 1999, p. 130). In other words, similar to Friere's comments that people who have systematically faced oppression are less likely to have expendable energy for fighting other people's oppressions, Oxhorn ponders whether it is victims who must now be held accountable for educating and assisting passive bystanders to make better pro-social choices. Rubin (1997) refers to this as a "one-directional notion of mobilization" (p. 131), in which it is assumed that poor people will unite in a single struggle against oppression. As several writers attest (Friere, 1970; Rubin, 1997; Oxhorn, 1999), this infers social contradictions that need to be explored.

Since 2010, the literature has focused on identifying the factors that act as barriers or facilitators in mobilizing bystanders to engage actively on behalf of an at-risk person. In other words, what helps bystanders become "upstanders" in support of victims? (Dominguez-Hernandez et al., 2018). On the one hand, a good relationship between the bystander and offender (siblings, friends) can be a barrier that favors passive behavior or inhibits the bystander from helping the victim. On the other hand, bonds of friendship between victims and bystanders encourage actions supporting the victims. Furthermore, in consideration of the social environments in which relationships between victims, perpetrators, and bystanders play out, theorists urge attention to the particular attitudes and behaviors to which members are expected to adhere, along with family expectations (DeSmet et al., 2016) and the perception of being cared for best within the family unit, fraught though family relationships might be. Passive bystanding is typical of cultures where collective interests outweigh individual harms such as some Asian cultures, and this is also typical of small collectivist communities that have learned to silence individual victims for the perceived greater good of the family in general. Researchers have concluded that these contextual factors are crucial in determining how or if victims may be saved from abuses and how practice, policy, and community educational planning may be developed to teach prosocial behavior. (DeSmet et al., 2012, 2014, 2016; Machackova et al., 2013).

Paolo Friere (1970) argued that when bystanders come from the same oppressive, violent communities as the victims, where they may have been violently victimized themselves, there manifests a deeply personal barrier to active intervention at the aid of another.

The oppressed, instead of striving for liberation, tend themselves to become oppressors, or "sub-oppressors." The very structure of their thought has been conditioned by the contradictions of the concrete, existential situation by which they were shaped. Their ideal is to be men, but for them, to be men is to be oppressors. This is their model of humanity.

(Freire, 1970, p. 45)

This quote directly relates to both Fanon and Jung's points of view, in which people who live within environments of oppression are not psychologically ready to be strong bystanders (psychoanalytical transformative learning). The societies have been constructed in accordance with patriarchal systems of control and dominance, in which bystanderism is an ethos more in keeping with victimization than with autonomy, as the SOSH has explained (social constructionism). In order to instigate radical change, a systemic plan needs to be developed and institutionalized, which will interrupt the power-based status quo and empower both victims and those who stand with victims to take pro-social, preventive action.

Mobilizing Bystanders Outside of the School Complex

The literature on bystander mobilization in situations of sexual abuse is mainly focused on preventing the harassment of children in schools and on college campuses in America. For example, Fischer et al. (2011) proposed that bystanders are more likely to intervene when a situation seems dangerous or physically life-threatening, as opposed to the shady, hidden, and silenced violence that defines sexual abuse, especially since victims of incest typically show no visible signs of having been violated. A "dangerous emergency", as Fischer would name it, is not usually recognized in cases of incest. This builds upon Darley and Latane's ground-breaking study (1970) on the bystander effect. They named five specific concerns in the minds of the bystanders that need to be resolved before definitive action is taken. Between 1970 and now, this five-step model has gained much traction, but for intervention in situations of incest, they show numerous gaps through which a child victim may fall un-helped (Darley & Latané, 1968; Latané & Nida, 1981).

One of these gaps manifests in step two, where interpreting a situation as an emergency is key to action. Fischer argued that unless a situation appears to be a "dangerous emergency," a bystander is unlikely to intervene, and CSA, as those in the field of child protection have seen, is generally silent and invisible. Another gap is at step five, which determines that the decision to take helping action relies upon the bystander not facing danger, legal battles, social or familial embarrassment, or aggressive retaliation. Reporting the abuse of a child victim almost always involves these things, and here is another big deterrent to mobilizing help.

In some jurisdictions, perpetrators may be punished by prison terms lasting up to 15 years. Therefore, where close friendships between perpetrators and bystanders exist, there is real hesitation to make a report. One wants their friend reprimanded and set back on the straight and narrow, but not necessarily imprisoned for a decade or two. Considerations also focus on financial support issues for the rest of the family if the main breadwinner (usually the male) is taken away.

Types of violence in the world are as diverse as they are troubling. From undocumented migrant workers escaping Haiti for the Dominican Republic with small children in tow to transgender sex workers smuggling themselves from Venezuela to Trinidad and Tobago, where income is better, but violence is perhaps more extreme, there are numerous different communities of vulnerable people facing acts of aggression within full view of silent others. Yet different collectives may contain spectators who, though appearing apathetic, may be fraught with complexity and the multiple layers of their wounds. Lest these collectives remain forever fated to the corruption of silenced spectatorship and a disintegrating responsibility to act, transformation must be mobilized.

References

Atienzo, E. E., Kaltenthaler, E., & Baxter, S. K. (2018). Barriers and facilitators to the implementation of interventions to prevent youth violence in Latin America: A systematic review and qualitative evidence synthesis. *Trauma, Violence & Abuse*, *19*(4), 420–430. https://doi.org/10.1177/152483801666404

Bar-On, D. (2001). The bystander in relation to the victim and the perpetrator: Today and during the Holocaust. *Social Justice Research*, *14*, 125–148. https://doi.org/10.1023/A:1012836918635

Blazquez, A., & Le Cour Grandmaison, R. (2021). Regional configurations of violence in Mexico: Accumulation, control and representation. *European Review of Latin American and Caribbean Studies*, *112*, 51–69. https://doi.org/10.32992/erlacs.10871

Chaney, C. (2020). Family stress and coping among African Americans in the age of COVID-19. *Journal of Comparative Family Studies*, *51*(3–4), 254–273. https://doi.org/10.3138/jcfs.51.3-4.003

Darley, J. M., & Latané, B. (1968). Bystander intervention in emergencies: Diffusion of responsibility. *Journal of Personality and Social Psychology*, *8*(4, Pt. 1), 377–383. https://doi.org/10.1037/h0025589

Decker, M. R., Wilcox, H. C., Holliday, C. N., & Webster, D. W. (2018). An integrated public health approach to interpersonal violence and suicide prevention and response. *Public Health Reports*, *133*(1_suppl), 65S–79S. https://doi.org/10.1177/0033354918800019

DeSmet, P., Cornillie, F., & Thorne, S. (2012). Digital games for language learning: challenges and opportunities [Special issue]. *ReCALL*, *24*, 243. https://doi.org/10.1017/S0958344012000134

DeSmet, A., Van Ryckeghem, D., Compernolle, S., Baranowski, T., Thompson, D., Crombez, G., Poels, K., Van Lippevelde, W., Bastiaensens, S., Van Cleemput, K., Vandebosch, H., & De Bourdeaudhuij, I. (2014, December). A meta-analysis of serious digital games for healthy lifestyle promotion. *Prev Med*, *69*, 95–107. https://doi.org/10.10.1016/j.ypmed.2014.08.026

DeSmet, A., Bastiaensens, S., Van Cleemput, K., Poels, K., Vandebosch, H., Cardon, G., et al. (2016). Deciding whether to look after them, to like it, or leave it: A multidimensional analysis of predictors of positive and negative bystander behavior in cyberbullying among adolescents. *Computers in Human Behavior*, *57*, 398–415. https://doi.org/10.1016/j.chb.2015.12.051

Dominguez-Hernandez, F., Bonell, L., & Martinez-Gonzales, A. (2018). A systematic literature review of factors that moderate bystanders' actions in cyberbullying. *Cyberpsychology: Journal of Psychosocial Research on Cyberspace*, *12*(4), Art. 1. https://doi.org/10.5817/CP2018-4-1

Evans, J. (2000). Globalisation: An annotated bibliography for the readers of *Assessment in Education. Assessment in Education: Principles, Policy and Practice*, *7*(3), 313–324. https://doi.org/10.1080/09695940050201325

Fischer, P., Krueger, J. I., Greitemeyer, T., Vogrincic, C., Kastenmüller, A., Frey, D., Heene, M., Wicher, M., & Kainbacher, M. (2011). The bystander-effect: A meta-analytic review on bystander intervention in dangerous and non-dangerous emergencies. *Psychological Bulletin*, *137*(4), 517–537. https://doi.org/10.1037/a0023304

Flecha, R. (2021). Second order sexual harassment: Violence against the silence break-ers who support the victims. *Violence Against Women*, *27*(11), 1980–1999. https://doi.org/10.1177/1077801220975495

Freire, P. (1970). *Pedagogy of the oppressed*. Continuum International Publishing Group.

Guiora, A. (2017). *The Crime of Complicity: The Bystander in the Holocaust*. American Bar Association.

Guiora, A. (2020). *Armies of Enablers: Survivor Stories of Complicity and Betrayal in Sexual Assaults*. American Bar Association.

Hilberg, R. (1997). The Goldhagen phenomenon. *Critical Inquiry*, *23*(4), 721–728. https://doi.org/10.1086/448851

Hulley, J., Bailey, L., Kirkman, G., Gibbs, G. R., Gomersall, T., Latif, A., & Jones, A. (2022). Intimate partner violence and barriers to help-seeking among black, Asian, minority ethnic and immigrant women: A qualitative metasynthesis of global research. *Trauma, Violence, & Abuse*, *24*(2), 1001–1015. https://doi.org/10.1177_15248380211050590

Jitman, L., & Machin, S. (2015). *Crime and violence in Latin America and the Caribbean: Towards evidence-based policies*. Centre Piece. https://cep.lse.ac.uk/pubs/download/cp461.pdf

Jones, A. D. (2021). Child sexual abuse as lifespan trauma within the context of intimate partner violence: Experiences of Caribbean women. *Frontiers in Sociology*, *6*. https://doi.org/10.3389/fsoc.2021.623661

Jones, A. D., Jemmott, E. T., Maharaj, P. E., & Breo, Da., H. (2014). An integrated systems model for preventing child sexual abuse. In: *An Integrated Systems Model for Preventing Child Sexual Abuse*. Palgrave Macmillan. https://doi.org/10.1057/9781137377661_1

Lacey, K. K., Jeremiah, R. D., & West, C. M. (2019). Domestic violence through a Caribbean lens: Historical context, theories, risks and consequences. *Journal of Aggression, Maltreatment & Trauma*, *30*(6), 761–780. https://doi.org/10.1080/10926771.2019.1660442

Latané, B., & Darley, J. M. (1970). *The Unresponsive Bystander: Why Doesn't He Help?* Appleton-Century-Crofts.

Machackova, H., Cerna, A., Sevcikova, A., Dedkova, L., & Daneback, K. (2013). Effectiveness of coping strategies for victims of cyberbullying. *Cyberpsychology: Journal of Psychosocial Research on Cyberspace*, *7*(3), Art. 5. https://doi.org/10.5817/CP2013-3-5

McBride, M. K., Carroll, M., Mellea, J. L., & Savoia, E. (2022). Targeted violence: A review of the literature on radicalization and mobilization. *Perspectives on Terrorism*, *16*(2), 24–38. https://doi.org/10.31235/osf.io/nw672

Moschella, E. A., & Banyard, V. L. (2020). Reactions to actions: Exploring how types of bystander action are linked to positive and negative consequences. *The Journal of Primary Prevention*, *41*(6), 585–602. https://doi.org/10.1007/s10935-020-00618-9

Flecha, R. (2021). Second order sexual harassment: Violence against the silence break-ers who support the victims. *Violence Against Women*, *27*(11), 1980–1999. https://doi.org/10.1177/1077801220975495

Latané, B., & Nida, S. (1981). Ten years of research on group size and helping. *Psychological Bulletin*, *89*(2), 308–324. https://doi.org/10.1037/0033-2909.89.2.308

Oxhorn, P. (1999). The ambiguous link: Social movements and democracy in Latin America. *Journal of Interamerican Studies and World Affairs*, *41*(3), 129–146. https://doi.org/10.2307/166161

Pérez, M. P., & Rasch, E. D. (2020). Resistance to hydropower developments in contexts of violence and organised crime in Mexico. *European Review of Latin American and Caribbean Studies/Revista Europea de Estudios Latinoamericanos y Del Caribe*, *110*, 123–143. https://www.jstor.org/stable/26979877

Polsky, S. (2022). Capital gains: Object ontologies, settler-colonialism, and financialized futures. In *The Dark Posthuman: Dehumanization, Technology, and the Atlantic World* (pp. 301–368). https://www.jstor.org/stable/j.ctv2x4kpwj

Rubin, J. W. (1997). *Decentering the Regime: Ethnicity, Radicalism, and Democracy in Juchitan, Mexico*. Duke University Press. https://doi.org/10.2307/j.ctv1220hrs

Salmivalli, C., Lagerspetz, K., Bjorkqvist, K., Osterman, K., & Kaukianen, A. (1996). Bullying as a group process: Participant roles and their relations to social status within the group. *Aggressive Behavior*, *2*(1), 1–15. https://doi.org/10.1002/(SICI)1098-2337(1996)22:1<1::AID-AB1>3.0.CO;2-T

Statista Research Department. (2022). *Latin America & Caribbean: Homicide rate 2021, by country*. https://www.statista.com/statistics/947781/homicide-rates-latin-america-caribbean-country

Wiesel, E. (1960). *Night*. Hill and Wang.

Wiesel, E. (2008). *The Night Trilogy: Night, Dawn, Day*. Hill and Wang.

Wiesel, E. (2011). *The Jews of Silence*. Schocken.

Zuckerhut, P. (2018). German and Mexican hegemonic constructions of masculinities and femininities in 19th century and its relevance in Mexico's twenty-first century's Feminicidio and Genocidio. *Anthropos*, *113*(2), 525–542. https://doi.org/10.5771/0257-9774-2018-2-525

Chapter 4

The Boy

He never knew what he had done wrong, but from that day on he began to be punished. Every day, after he arrived home from school and ate a delicious supper with the other children in the house, he would receive his punishment. Then, he would shower, wash the evidence of his punishment away, and get into bed with a book. For years, Yusuf thought hard about what he was doing to deserve such treatment. He even asked the man, "What did I do? At least tell me what I did so wrong!" but the man never responded with more than grunts, snorts, and harder thrashings. The man went where he wanted, did what he pleased, and spoke a language of pure force, while Yusuf learned to be perpetually alert in case he needed to jump out of the way of the blow that was coming. The blow was just as often psychic as it was physical, and it was always sexual, too.

One of the other boys, Selim, was in the same boat, but you couldn't get confirmation from him. "You stay where you are there!" Selim told him. "You hold your own corner! Study yourself! Mind your business!" Drool slipped down Yusuf's chin. Snot ran from his nose. The night staff said the boy was peeing on his bed again, something he had grown out of years before. Worse, his underpants were always stained with leaked feces, and the nurses threatened to rub his nose in it like a dog.

One afternoon, when the man took all of the residents hiking and looked down from the top of the cliff he had scaled to beckon at the boy, the boy first looked around to make sure he was the only one being beckoned and then blurted out, "Nah! After he done with me up there, I will never be able to come back down!" The boy began to shake so violently that he let go of all his water. The bottle of water in his hand, the spit that collected in his mouth, and the urine in his bladder; he let it all go and then let himself go too, falling to the ground with terrible shakings. "Oh God, Lord!" The chaperone shouted, "He's taking a fit! The boy is having a seizure!"

That was only the first of many such fits, and they continued with such frequency and severity that the boy was moved into the female chaperone's room to sleep at night. She became his keeper and guarded him against catching fits where no one could see him and banging his brains out on the floor. In the months and years to come, the boy thought back to the first incident and tried to figure out the cause,

DOI: 10.4324/9781003223603-6

but the only images that returned to his mind were the man's long, beckoning finger curling at him from above and him beginning to leak from every orifice.

In this residential facility, in the administration's wisdom, they had confiscated photographs of the children's parents and families. They believed that since the children had come from abusive, neglectful, and abandoning homes, it would serve them no good to have visual reminders. The administration opted for the annihilation of memory, "fresh starts", and "new beginnings", but in the void that this depersonalization created and with darkly shrouded memories never erased but repressed and haunting, the boy found symbolisms representing the one crisp reality that he did know. The man's long, curling finger became the recurring image that populated his nightmares and tortured ruminations.

"It's inside me", he would sob to the keeper when he woke up shivering at night. "It's inside me. It's taking me". These simple, straightforward words, this crystal-clear cry for help, were instantly misinterpreted as possession by a demonic force.

Additionally, when specifically asked of the boy, "Do you believe you are possessed by something inside of you?" he answered, "Yes", and the institution's external counselor checked a box. "Do you hear it talking to you? Do you hear its voice?" Shivering and shaking at the edge of his bed, the boy said "yes". "Does it tell you to do things that you feel you have to obey?" The boy nodded hard and opened his mouth in an awful wail. "I can't take it again", he cried. The counselor checked all the boxes in her repertoire of symptoms, snapped her file shut, and whispered to the keeper as she left the room. The boy could not hear what she said, but he didn't get a comforting feeling.

The counselor would have called herself efficient, certainly, and her superiors would have agreed. But she had been trained along the lines of encouraging psychosocial functionality, keeping positive to avoid anxiety and depression, and meeting sociocultural expectations. As for working with minds that had suffered sufficient trauma to crack them open, the counselor was content to simply diagnose a psychotic break with reality, including seeing things, hearing voices, paranoia, and "fits". She pronounced the condition a terminal mental disease like cancer and, therefore, beyond the scope of her practice.

Martín-Baró described this common approach to treating mental health conditions as psychology's cleaving to the early natural sciences, with lab coats, instruments, and no concept of relationality to the subject. Theirs was a pseudo-militant approach, defined by methods, measurements, and an objective to unearth the "truth" about a client. In the early days, this was considered a developed medical psychology, but in the case of Yusuf, for one, it left the patient unseen, cold, suspicious, and unhelped. As Fanon later wrote, the idea of looking at mental health from the point of view of the patient rather than the practitioner had not occurred. In fact, if a patient shared their experiences in a manner that was looked at suspiciously by the culture, the patient's issue was generally dismissed or redefined in terms that best suited the practitioner's understanding.

In retrospect, Yusuf's fits could be diagnosed as psychogenic blackouts, which are described as psychogenic nonepileptic seizures (PNES) caused by trauma and distress. According to the American Academy of Family Physicians (AAFP) (2005), these are "episodes of movement, sensation, or behaviors that are similar to epileptic seizures but do not have a neurological origin; rather, they are somatic manifestations of psychological distress" (pp. 849–856). While the AAFP lists substance use, movement disorders, and cardiac arrhythmias as potential causal factors, many patients have a history of sexual or physical abuse.

PNES has been in the world since the late 1800s when French neurologist Jean-Martin Charcot first described it as "epileptiform hysteria". Freud later coined the term "conversion hysteria", in which the physical symptoms represented an attempt by the unconscious to communicate unbearable psychic conflicts often related to sex. PNES has a prevalence of 2–33 cases per 100,000 (2023), and given its rarity, in small rural communities like the one in which Yusuf's residential home was established, counselors were not always up to par with rare psychological conditions. This home's counselor contented herself by identifying Yusuf entirely with the idea that he had himself declared; that he was possessed, and she left it at that. Rather, she referred her patient to prayer. Like many mental health practitioners, hers was a hermeneutics of suspicion. She took a punitive stance regarding irregular behaviors among the child population, and this orientation was a normalized factor of this entire institution's *weltanschauung*.

In Jung's approach to phenomenology, he urges clinicians not to be in such a rush to diagnose and prescribe. Instead, clinicians are urged to lean into the precise words or images clients provide on their own terms in a non-reductive manner. As Brooks reports, "Jung (1941) explicitly warns us against looking too soon for explanation … as explanations may lead away from the meaning that is immanent" (Brooks, 2015, p. 33).

The International Hearing Voices Movement is relatively new globally, established by Romme and Escher in 1987. It is a conglomeration of organizations and individuals challenging the notion that auditory and verbal hallucinations are necessarily a symptom of mental illness. Instead, they regard hearing voices as understandable, meaningful, and somewhat "normal", given a person's life history. They report that over 70% of voice hearers have previously suffered severely traumatic or intensely emotional events or faced an event that activated the memory of an earlier trauma (Romme & Escher, 2013). As such, they are much more than emissions from a damaged brain. Romme and Escher's theory proposed that there is a high correlation between voice hearing and abuse in children and that some people who hear voices have a deep need to talk to others about it without being stigmatized as mad, or as possessed. However, in the same way that knowledge of Psychogenic Non-Epileptic Seizures had not found its way into Yusuf's community of practitioners, neither had this new approach to hearing voices, such as the voice that Yusuf reported.

Yusuf now developed the habit of holding onto his ears, blocking sound. He looked downwards all the time, blocking sight. He lost track of what stimuli came from the outside or inside, whether he was perceiving a material truth or having hallucinations. His sensory floor had been completely shaken; its walls blasted apart. He left his mouth to hang open and let drool leak, and when the other boys in the home teased his schizoid appearance, he reacted with violent intensity, like a cornered dog. These tantrums earned him further predictable punishments from the man. Yusuf could hear his belt unbuckling from a mile away, and he came to believe that the man deliberately orchestrated provocations against him, causing his all too visible buttons to get pushed and exploded so the man could pounce on him and justify the abuses that continued in a repetitive cycle for years.

The boy began to take fits at school. In the middle of the chemistry lab, he would fall backward off the stool to smash his head on the concrete floor. Selim preferred to think of Yusuf as "taking" a fit, as opposed to having a fit or catching a fit, because Selim believed he helped himself to them purposefully. Moreover, the boy screamed out sometimes, leaning forward and down as if to direct the sound into his own body, to use sound to drive out something lodged there. It was spine-chilling, came from out of the blue, and would end as randomly as it started. They said his soul had been invaded and devoured, and the boy agreed. "Yes, by a curly finger", he said, "And by the sound of an unbuckling belt".

Guardians, teachers, and church people took up a collection and sent the boy away to get an MRI, but finding nothing medically wrong with him, then sent him to priests to chase the demons away. This is a form of exorcism, as Rahimi writes (2021), in which the possessing spirits are seen as destructive, polluting, or pathogenic. It is the job of the pastor to extract them out of a body and lure them off on another path.

"How are you? Are you all right?" Selim asked him when he came back. "I've gone missing", the boy answered. "I seem to have gone missing. I wish I was here". The boy developed a mercurial way of talking and moving, slipping and sliding from one state of non-being to another. He avoided visibility and kept his head low, walking in a skulking, slouching manner and treading like a cat.

No professional, not even the well-meaning ones, could relate to what was going on behind the closed doors of this institutional home, especially since it was meant to be a helping place rather than a nest of evil, at least in the case of the one chosen boy.

Psychologists work with evil all the time, helping victims of beatings, rape, and torture, along with more subtle abuses like hatred and indifference. Occasionally, we work with perpetrators of evil as well. Yet, as professionals, we are wont to shy away from the term *evil*, having been mis-educated into accepting that it is non-scientific or subjective. This creates a blind spot for psychologists, which may then be filled by unskilled practitioners from either religion or psychology, which is all the more likely when the client is impoverished, low in education, black, or from another marginalized population. To mention that you feel yourself spirit possessed is to put yourself at the bottom of the mainstream psychological barrel.

Psychiatry, Psychosis-Like Experiences (PLEs) and Possession Syndrome

It is my position that shamans – individuals trained in accordance with Indigenous beliefs and practices, may be as highly skilled as academics who are generally trained exclusively in the Western medical model. I even argue in favor of a strong practice similarity in some modalities. Of course, the opposite is also true: academic psychologists may be as poorly trained as incompetent practitioners in any field.

C. G. Jung visited East Africa to study the inner life of the people there and to confer with their traditional healers (Jung, 1973, pp. 255–256). He similarly befriended a Pueblo Chief and wrote introductions to translations of the Tibetan Book of the Dead and the seminal Taoist text, The Secret of the Golden Flower. Being heavily invested in inter-cultural contexts, Jungian psychology helps us hold all possibilities of psychic movement as equally meaningful. While many psychiatrists find it difficult to relate to the spiritual beliefs of their patients, Jungian psychology provides a framework for non-judgemental reception of all the diverse phenomena, purely as they arise.

Jung has wide popular appeal in diverse populations like Italy, Brazil, Australia, and South Africa, as well as in many parts of Latin America and the Spanish Caribbean. However, as I discuss in the chapter on Nile, the English-speaking Caribbean has thus far avoided the uptake of Jung and his psychoanalytical movement.

Comas Diaz wrote (quote from Abramovich & Kirmayer, 2003, p. 160):

> As a Puerto Rican, I had encountered ethnic discrimination among dynamically oriented psychotherapists and was suspicious of a therapeutic orientation that did not examine itself along those lines. I chose a Jungian analyst instead, finding this orientation less dogmatic and more receptive to cultural diversity … The psychotherapeutic journey was nurturing, liberating, and actualizing. Combining my long-standing interest in mythology and tradition helped me further integrate spiritual principles into my psychotherapy practice.

When any disciplined mental health worker refuses to acknowledge manifestations of evil, this leaves clients who believe themselves to be victims of evil or possessed by evil to perhaps search among the habitats of shady practitioners for deliverance from their psychic or somatic suffering. Often, these untrained counselors do more harm than good; worse, they turn patients away from the authentic assistance they need.

Refusing to acknowledge that some cultures believe in human possession by spirits (which is not the same as believing in superstitions or the supernatural), be they evil or good, creates other blind spots and failed opportunities for sound psychological work. Hussein Rassool, a professor of Islamic psychology, wrote that in the Muslim community because it is widely accepted that *Jinn* spirits can cause mental illness in humans, psychologists are called upon to acquire advanced differential diagnostic skills to be able to offer help to those who believe themselves thus afflicted (Rassool, 2018).

In 1994, the Diagnostic and Statistical Manual (DSM), produced by the American Psychological Association and currently in its 5th edition, added a new diagnostic category, "Religious or Spiritual Problems". The section invites professionals to respect patients' beliefs and rituals. However, because exact criteria are not outlined, the category is left open to speculation, with most mainstream psychiatrists and other mental health professionals projecting personal distinctions upon what is "normal" and what is "pathological" or "delusional". In 2013, the DSM further updated itself to include the concept of "culture-bound syndrome" or "cultural idioms of distress" (p. 758).

Pierre (2001) refers to "entire delusional subcultures" and "religious beliefs that exist outside of the scientific domain", which, of course, is a derogatory manner of looking at the issue. This perspective derives from an old Freudian position; Freud having been an atheist who referred to religion as a universal obsessional neurosis. Other cognitive behavioral psychologists similarly claimed a *causal* relationship between religion and psychosis. This leaves the way open for practitioners who cleave to very colonized understandings of psychology to express disrespect and disregard for clients wanting to discuss notions of possession by spirits.

However, according to Jung, within the psyche, there are disturbances that may overwhelm a person in surprising ways. "They are the gremlins and inner demons that may catch a person by surprise … and are differentiated from disturbances brought about by stressors originating in the external environment, even though they may and often do relate intimately to one another" (Stein, p. 40).

More recent scholarship in the field of psychiatry accepts the view that religious beliefs are not to be considered delusional if they are culturally normal since the function of belief is itself social and not purely epistemic. Sofou et al. (2021) wrote of the clinical importance of investigations of religiosity in patients with psychotic disorders. Most importantly, Sofou et al. (2021) agree that the content of religious delusions is significantly influenced by the beliefs and attitudes of the patient's immediate family and cultural environments.

In the Caribbean and Latin America, as well as among Muslim and Indigenous populations everywhere, explanatory models of illness, coping mechanisms, and help-seeking behaviors may extend past the Western biopsychosocial approach to include multifactorial influences such as possession syndrome. Some believe that in the etiology of illness, the supernatural world, including God, ancestor spirits, witchcraft, or sorcery, may be seen as the agents behind mental illness as a form of punishment for wrongdoing or sin. In a 2008 study about global perceptions of mental illness, 84% of respondents believed in the devil's possession of mentally ill persons (Abu-Ras & Abu-Bader, 2008). Respondents scoring similarly highly included diverse populations like Swedish Somalis (Johnsdotter et al., 2011) and South African healers and psychiatrists (Ally & Laher, 2008).

It is important that health care professionals have an awareness of this … in order to provide culturally congruent and appropriate care and management.

(Rassool, 2018, p. 4)

In Yusuf's case, he was neither demon-possessed nor did he have a psychosis originating in organic brain dysfunction. However, he had reported on the contents of his nightmares as they had had a shattering impact on him. *Interpretations* about the content of his dreams came from his keeper and the institution's mental health personnel, who misread the symptomatology arising from child abuse psychosis.

This is a serious mistake for voice-hearers with backgrounds of child abuse psychosis. According to Manuel Gonzales De Chaves, Professor and Chief of the Psychiatric Service of General University Hospital (Romme et al., 2013):

> (There are) some serious consequences for the diagnoses, image, and stigmatization of insanity for all those who, with whatever frequency, intensity and attitude, had the subjective experience of hearing voices at some time in their lives.
>
> (De Chaves, as cited in Romme, et al, 2013, p. xv)

Raising the awareness of mental health professionals on issues of a religious and spiritual nature can be beneficial in both preventing and treating psychotic disorders (Sofou et al., 2021).

There is also a racist inequity and other multilayered factors affecting Yusuf's care and treatment. He is small, black, relatively impoverished, abandoned by his family, sexually abused by the administrative head, and then Yusuf began to abuse others in turn. He was called "retard" due to the somatization of his deteriorating psychological condition. Finally, he originates in the tropical rain forest, where mainstream institutions do not usually give indigenous peoples' religious beliefs credence. In the interplay between the boy's culture of origin, the culture of the institution itself, and the culture of the clinicians, the child client was the loser all around. In Fanon's framework, he was fully othered, and as Toni Morrison wrote:

> For humans as an advanced species, our tendency to separate and judge those not in our clan as enemies but as the vulnerable and deficient needing control has a long history.
>
> (Morrison, 2017, p. 3)

Nowhere is this controlling separation more evident than in our treatment of individuals with mental health issues, even if those have arisen because of victimization as a child. According to Jung, the actions we take as individuals and members of our cultural group reflect an unconscious motivation. Jung defines the cultural or collective unconscious as containing all of the psychic contents belonging to a society, a people, or humankind. This comprises not only concepts but also feelings.

In a recent study, Petti et al. (2023) found that marginalized racial groups are at a more elevated risk for racial discrimination and trauma. This is a likely contributory factor to the reasons why Black/African Americans, as well as Latin American, Caribbean, and Asian peoples, tend to stay away from formal mental health care services. One may understand this phenomenon when individuals travel to foreign places. However when clients are marginalized by professionals born and raised in the same margins with the same multicultural roots is deeply disappointing. This has to do with the blind acceptance of imported Western concepts and practices wholesale, without regard for cultural adaptations and sensitivities, as Martin-Baro and Fanon have both made so clear.

As for Yusuf, several times abandoned, without psychological care, and with unbearable tensions running through his body, he began to hurt and violate others as a means of psychic release. Boy or girl, there was no difference to him. It only mattered that they were smaller than him, both physically and intellectually, so he could exert some measure of dominance for once in his life. As Fanon wrote, "The colonized man will first manifest the aggressiveness which has been deposited in his bones, against his own people" (Fanon, 1967, p. 40).

Jung has written of *Ergriffenheit*, a state of being seized or possessed. The term postulates not only an Ergriffener (one who is seized) but also an Erfreifer (one who seizes) (Dohe, 2011). Alternatively, as it may be read, victim turned perpetrator.

This is by no means to suggest that all male perpetrators were themselves violated first. A 2013 United Nations research study on violence by men against women found that:

> Out of 10,000 men surveyed, one-half reported the use of physical and/or sexual violence against a woman, and one-quarter of those surveyed admitted to rape. The most common motivation that men cited for committing rape was sexual entitlement – a belief that men have a right to have sex with women regardless of consent.
>
> (W.H.O., 2013)

Jacques Derrida, who formulated his notion of "hauntology" in contrast to the traditional "ontology", speaks of the *specter,* such as the depersonalized boy, as no longer having any being in itself, but still suffering the "traumatic compulsion to repeat; a structure that repeats, a fatal pattern" (Fisher, 2009, p. 19)

"The desire to dominate when he himself was dominated was strong and instinctive and belonged to the unquellable depths of himself" (Alexis, 2015, p. 62)

This may also be read as yet another type of "possession" by a powerful, negative father complex, as we have seen in the cases of Carrie and Melanie. With Yusuf, he unconsciously co-opted the monstrous habits of the primary father figure in his life – the man at the head of the residential facility. According to Jung, an inner perpetrator develops when a child is treated badly or abusively. In my practice, I have very often seen this manifest in women of middle age, who report "hearing voices" of past abusive or dysfunctional parents jeering at their "stupidity", "blackness", and other terms intended to insult and demean them. Especially offensive, for example, is the mother who lives with a simmering rage against an experience of rape that occurred during her adolescence, and often, publicly (even on social media) refers to the child who was conceived during that incident as "a rape child". Needless to say, this trajectory produces an internalized victimization in which the child grows up to believe and act in the manner they were raised. We saw this in the case of Melanie, too, in which the habits of parental bullying, abuse, and gaslighting become potent directives for the child to unconsciously follow.

If there is a psychosis, the hearing of voices is often no more than the ongoing tyrannical influence, or possession, of the abuser, as the incestuous father inhabited or possessed his child victim in the case of Carrie.

Like Fanon, Paolo Freire taught that seeking escape from oppressive situations is merely a beginning. The deep psychological revolution must include freeing ourselves from the piece of the oppressor that possesses us and embeds within us. As Audre Lorde (2007) put it, "the piece of the oppressor which knows only the oppressor's tactics, the oppressor's relationships." (p. 123).

Yusuf always made his victims eat food first, providing nurturing in the way he had received it. Food was the one good constancy in Yusuf's life. Staff at the home were not trained or credentialed childcare providers; the institution had no funding to attract such professionals. Nor were they necessarily kind, as many of them resented that these children had come from lowly backgrounds and were now elevated by their very lowliness to positions that demanded more attention than the carers themselves had ever received. But there was always food. Split peas soup served on Saturdays at lunch was Yusuf's favorite. Week after week, the soup remained exactly the same. The same spoonful of salt, a cupful of coconut milk, pigtails, Irish potatoes, onions, and thyme. The cook brooked no deviation from her established recipe, and the children were her happy beneficiaries. One might say that it was into that big pot that she consistently poured all her love. In soup, Yusuf trusted.

When administering the food he gave to others, Yusuf spoke soft, reassuring words. As he opened wounds in boys smaller than himself, he looked deeply into their eyes, curious to excavate how feelings ought to be felt. He had no more feelings of his own, you see, except for a pervasive sense of loneliness, despair, and a compulsion to repeat. Try as he might, he was unable to connect with anything that felt substantial in himself, so he crept on others, imitating their looks, sounds, and responses. He searched out other lost children in his village and gathered them into the arms of "love". He curled his finger at them, and they came. When he violated them after showing them "love", they responded not with anger and resistance but with confusion. The confusion kept them silent, trying in vain to figure things out.

Jung's Typology, the Sensing Function, and Child Victims of Abuse

I have found Jung's typology extremely useful to an understanding of the impact of over-sexualization or hyper-sexualization of small children, particularly on a cumulative basis. Typology does not specifically address itself either to child abuse or to states that resemble possession, either of an emotional or spiritual nature.

Nevertheless, Jung's typology represents his first presentation of his unique psychological ideas to the world in his 1921 book Psychological Types. This first book followed upon his first official scholarly publication, his doctoral study, on the Psychology and Pathology of So-Called Occult Phenomena. Following this, Jung introduced his newly discovered feature of unconscious processes, which he named "complexes", and produced another book that took up two burning psychiatric problems of the day, psychosis and schizophrenia, in the Psychology of Dementia Praecox.

Over 100 years later, these central problems continue to wrestle with us. It is to Jung's theories on "so-called occult phenomena", personal and cultural complexes, archetypal patterns, the unconscious, and psychosis to which I turn in an attempt to describe how child victims of sexual abuse develop child abuse psychosis, which more often than not is misunderstood, misdiagnosed and therefore insufficiently treated.

Jung's system of typology specifically helps when working with the different qualities of sensations and feelings that run amok in a child's small body when the child is sexually violated. It provides vivid insight into what transpires when so much sensory data starts rushing through an immature brain, which in turn points the way to the quality of response necessary to guide healing.

Typology is a theory of personality development. Jung's initial motivation for investigating typology was his need to understand why Freud and Adler's individual personalities led them to view neurosis so differently. Where Freud saw his patients as being preeminently dependent upon and defined in relation to significant external objects (extraverted sensing), Adler's emphasis was on how a person, or subject, seeks its own security and supremacy (introverted sensing). In my view, similarly to how patients with bipolar disorder will cycle between one opposite mood and another, sometimes in relatively quick succession, so will a child victim of sexual abuse, under a flood of activated sensory data, move with similar psychic dynamism. The child will "become complexed" and either turn radically inward (as in the case of Yusuf) or outward (as in the case of Vladimir) depending upon the trigger and circumstances of the perceived threat or flashback. The delusions that make-up a part of the check list for psychosis or schizophrenia, may instead be based on some kind of sensory experience that a victim of sexual abuse has suffered.

When Vincent Van Gogh wrote to describe his experience of psychosis when he was hospitalized in 1888, he chose to reference his sensing function. He described the sensation of anguish, called *Voir-Rouge*, from which certain of his "companions in misfortune" frequently suffered (Bailey, 2022).

Like Carrie, Yusuf was never able to loosen the grip in which his conditioned sensory reflexes held him. Both body and mind had been made unstable at too young an age for equilibrium to fully return without targeted intervention.

Writing on Jung, Daryl Sharp said, "Jung suspected there might be physiological causes of which we have as yet no precise knowledge since a reversal or distortion of type often proves harmful to one's physical well-being" (Sharp, 1987, p. 27).

Jung wrote, "As a rule, whenever such a fabrication of type takes place, the individual becomes neurotic later and can be cured only by developing the attitude consonant with his nature" (Jung, CW 6, 1976, p. 560).

With child victims of sexual abuse, the child's response to the object (abuser) is usually conditioned by the object (in the case of extraverted sensing), resulting in a developing personality that seeks out objects, both people and situations, that excite the strongest sensations. They develop a strong, sensuous tie to the external world. Jung wrote: "Objects are valued in so far as they excite sensations, and, so far as lies within the power of sensation, they are fully accepted into conscientiousness whether they are compatible with rational judgments or not" (Jung, 1976, CW 6, p 605).

Adult Extraverted Sensation types are wont to be impeccably mannered in fashion, aesthetics, and cuisine situations. Jung describes this type as having "lively capacity ... and very good company" (CW 6, par. 605). But for the child victim struggling to catch themselves during a sexual assault by an adult whose intention is to annihilate the self-agency of their victim, orientation toward that external object becomes a battle for life over death with psychological complexities that are far too over-whelming for child minds to make any real sense of. Only sensation remains, driving the victim to orient themselves from that "lost in the sensory forest" place that I described in the chapter on Carrie, perpetually thereafter being "desirous of the strongest sensations, and these, by his very nature, he can only receive from outside" (Jung, 1976, CW 6, par. 607).

In its full quaternity, Jung's typology includes other functions that balance us out, as each human being contains a measure of all, though one is normally dominant. For sex abuse victims, however, the psychological situation becomes pathological.

Regarding the Introverted Sensing type, the description given by von Franz is even more fitted to child victims of chronic abuse who learn to hyper-analyze every situation and person for signs of danger lurking. She wrote:

> When somebody comes into the room, such a type notices the way the person comes in, the hair, the expression on the face, the clothes, and the way the person walks ... every detail is absorbed. The impression comes from the object to the subject; it is as though a stone falls into deep water – the impression falls deeper and deeper and sinks in. Outwardly, the introverted sensation type looks utterly stupid. He just sits and stares, and you do not know what is going on within him. He looks like a piece of wood with no reaction at all ... but inwardly, the impression is being absorbed.
>
> (von Franz & Hillman, 2013, pp. 27–28)

Psychiatry generally understands psychosis and schizophrenia to be disorders of thought or thinking. Schizophrenia, in fact, translates (in German) as a splitting of the various parts of the thought process. However, we can see from Jung's descriptions that sensory input can also be mis-sorted and misinterpreted by the person herself. Furthermore, ferreting out an appropriate response to the flood of sensory input that accompanies sexual abuse, is well beyond the capacity of a child.

To consider the issue from an adult's perspective, two male survivors of child sexual abuse shared these experiences:

I was about three or four years old and playing underneath the house when the gardener came in and grabbed me from the back. "Don't make noise", he told me, "Hush your mouth". I could hear my grandmother walking around upstairs looking for me. She started calling my name, but I felt powerless to respond. The gardener heard her, too, so he started hurrying up. He had me bent over a piece of wall and I felt him drag down my short pants. When I looked behind to see what he was doing, all I could see was a huge pink penis with an eye. I realize it could not have been that big, but to me then it looked bigger than I was. He had one hand in the front of me, rubbing my groin, and he started pushing his hips into my bum. I realized he was going to put that big penis inside of me, and I still could not call out. My grandmother was calling me more urgently and I still cannot fully explain the rush of sensations I experienced but I was overwhelmed. Terror, curiosity, arousal, fear, my heart was pounding in my head. I badly wanted to run, to scream for my Granny, to kick at that man, but I was frozen. Then Granny's head appeared at the window, and she could see my little face looking up. "There you are!" she called. "What are you doing there? Lunch is getting cold!" Just as the gardener fit his penis to my bum, he dropped me and disappeared. I never said a word to anyone, but all through my life, even now, when I'm a grown married man, whenever I get into a sexual situation, I feel ashamed. I feel like racing away. I cheat a lot on my wife, and she calls me a sex addict, but no, I am simply looking for someone who might make me feel differently this time. I haven't yet found the one. I am drinking heavily these days, and that is why I am in therapy. To stop the drinking.

I was in my first year of college, about 18 years old when a female teacher called me into her office and raped me. I know it sounds ridiculous. But she was my favorite teacher. When she hugged me up and started kissing my neck, I felt bad to shove her away. She had her hand on my penis and it was responding, so she was laughing thinking I was excited but I was horrified. She was not good looking and she was old. Here I was, a young athlete, saving myself for a lovely young girl one day who I would love, like in the movies. The teacher was nothing like I had in mind for my first time. She climbed in my lap and had sex with me, and I didn't do anything. I felt disgusted with myself. Up to today, now that I have a girlfriend I love, I can't get stimulated unless she kind of forces me. Not unless she treats me rough and dominates me. Then I get aroused. But my girlfriend's personality is not like that. She is a sweet, quiet girl. My relationship is getting messed up. My whole life is just messed up.

The difference between pornography and healthy, consensual sexual engagement is also a good illustration of the issue. Pornography (and forced sex) is a direct denial of sexuality as it is focused on the suppression of true feelings. Pornography privileges sensation without feeling, whereas a healthy relationship represents the highest sense of self and draws forward our strongest feelings. As Audre Lorde wrote, "Having experienced the fullness of this depth of feeling and recognizing its power, in honor and self-respect, we can require no less of ourselves" (Lorde, p. 54).

Systems of typology have been in the world from the time of the ancient Asian astrologers and later in the time of the physiological typology of Greek medicine. Jung's model, which he developed after 20 years of research in the fields of psychopathology, practical psychology, philosophy, mythology, and literature, was mainly concerned with the movement of psychic energy. I relate this to the sensory energies moving in child victims of sexual abuse, which naturally and easily lend to appearing demon possessed as in the case of Yusuf, or to psychotic break down either at the time or later in their lives as with Carrie and Melanie.

In Jung's model, along with the two "attitudes" of Extraversion and Introversion, there is a quaternity of Thinking, Feeling, Sensation, and Intuition. Each of these four is required for comprehensive self-understanding. No one is better than the other, but any one of them, depending on the individual and his circumstance, will become dominant or more prominently differentiated.

In the case of CSA, the Sensation function is forced into primacy. Sensation establishes that something exists. Along with Intuition, Sensation is an "illogical" function that operates independently of reason. Intuition picks up (phenomenologically) what exists in the inside world, while Sensation records what is taken in by sight, taste, touch, and so on. As Jung very importantly said, "Judgement cannot keep pace with experience" (Jung, CW6, par. 371). Jung writes:

> The demands of society compel a man to apply himself first and foremost to the differentiation of the function with which he is best equipped by nature or which will secure him the greatest social success. Very frequently, indeed, as a general rule.
>
> (Jung, CW6, par. 763)

Repetition Compulsion

Repetition compulsion is a psychological phenomenon in which an individual unconsciously repeats past traumatic experiences in an attempt to gain mastery over them. This concept was first articulated by Freud, who believed that a person's inability to squarely face past traumatic events in the light of present, transformative awareness, coupled with the human tendency to seek comfort in the familiar, leads us to "the desire to return to an earlier state of things". This tendency can manifest in various dysfunctional ways, such as self-destructive behavior, seeking out abusive relationships as a means of fixing the abuse that happened in the past, and becoming a perpetrator when one has experienced violence as a child. It is a literal though unconscious reenactment of the abuse, a means of gaining mastery over the original sense of utter powerlessness. Victims feel wronged but feel justified in returning that wrong to others. People filled with hate because of things a parent did twenty, thirty, forty years ago can (perhaps unconsciously) extract revenge from everyone who tries to get close

> Adults, as well as children, often feel compelled to re-create the moment of terror, either in literal or disguised form. People reenact the traumatic moment with a fantasy of changing the outcome of the dangerous encounter. In their attempts to undo the traumatic moment, survivors may even put themselves at risk of further harm.
>
> (Hermann,1987)

Unfortunately, when the pattern of abuse is repeated, the victim is generally re-victimized and may feel doubly doomed. However, the repetition is, in fact, re-occurring due to their own unconscious choices. Self-worth is thus diminished even more, and the cycle continues. Note that behaviors in the context of adult relationships with non-abusive partners may nevertheless draw out self-hatred, hostility, and detachment or dissociation as other forms of repetition compulsion. This is unfortunately an issue that I see very often in couples counseling.

> Adults, as well as children, often feel compelled to re-create the moment of terror, either in literal or disguised forms. People re-enact the traumatic moment with a fantasy of changing the outcome of the dangerous encounter. In their attempts to undo the traumatic moment, survivors may even put themselves at risk of further harm.
>
> (Judith Herman)

But returning to Yusuf, why would he find himself stuck in a cycle of repetition compulsion? Simply (although it is certainly not simple but a deep and sinister psychological complex), in order to face the worst demons he had ever known, he challenged them once again, and this time, he made sure to come out the victor due to his superior and aggressive domination of the situation. This archetypal need is found in the wisdom of indigenous tribes where each and every young man, with elders as learned, able, and loving guides, is put through a period of initiation in which they are tested to their limits, provided with all the teachings and tools that they need to survive, and finally welcomed back home to the village triumphant, having bested the lion, so to speak. They are perhaps scarred and battered but stronger in spirit and ready for adulthood. Without these healthy traditional rites of passage, children like Yusuf are left prey to the meandering "demonic" forces among us, generally of human form and desire.

To press the metaphor that makes sense to me, if one becomes lost in a forest, for example, a first objective is often to return to the location where one last recognized him or herself or the surroundings, a point of reference, and to begin tracking from there. Child victims of rape often inadvertently, illogically, orient themselves from the incident of rape to try to catch a sense of bearing from when they last felt strong, innocent, and pure. That is, just before the first violation. Tragically, the sensory impetus to recover power and direction sometimes leads to repetition compulsion.

Yusuf's path took a new turn when spontaneously he began to dream of a figure he identified as God, but this God wore a big skirt, had a bosom and a wide lap into which she gathered the boy to hold him and rock him and cause a great tsunami of warm, soothing kindness to wash him with nameless emotion. He imagined he heard singing. He dreamed this same dream frequently, up to several times in one night. Jung wrote about an archetypal experience he'd had when he was 12 years old.

> I was taking the long road to school from Klein-Huningen, where we lived, to Basel, when suddenly, for a single moment, I had the overwhelming impression of having just emerged from a dense cloud. I knew all at once: now I am *myself*! It was as if a wall of mist were at my back, and behind that wall, there was not yet an "I". But, at this moment, *I came upon myself…* Previously, I had been willed to do this and that; now, *I* willed. This experience seemed to me tremendously important and new: there was "authority" in me.
>
> (Gulick, 1981)

At another time during his childhood (circa, 1913), Jung experienced a figure coming to him in his dreams. He named this figure Philemon. He considered Philemon his prime teacher about "the reality of the psyche", a being of superior insight, and Jung engaged him in active imagination for years to come.

Based on personal experiences and those of his clients, Jung proposed that in the absence of an able human guide, an inner companion or ally appears in dreams. Through active imagination within a therapeutic encounter, one then has the opportunity to expand upon the appearance of this imaginal being and find a unique guiding and protective figure.

Archetypal Psychology

As mentioned before, regarding the dark goddess Melinoe, Jung began researching and writing about archetypes during his work with people with schizophrenia at the Burgholzli Hospital in 1919. He defined archetypes as primordial images, an inborn form of intuition (Jung, CW, vol. 8, para 277). Archetypes arise from the collective unconscious, inherited from previous generations and extending back to the earliest days of human experience. They are not dependent on individual experience and are formed beyond the level of conscious awareness. The formal discipline of Archetypal Psychology developed as a post-Jungian movement in the early 1970s under the guidance of James Hillman, the first director of the Jung Institute in Zurich.

Victor Frankl, a psychiatrist, wrote of the interrelationship between psychotherapy and theology in several of his 20 books, including Psychotherapy and Existentialism (1967), The Will to Meaning (1970), Man's Search for Meaning (1973), and Man's Search for Ultimate Meaning (2000). Also, a phenomenologist, Frankl, proposed that an "unconscious God", that is, the presence of God arising unexpectedly and unbidden from our unconscious, may happen "even in cases of severe mental illness" (Frankl, 2000, p. 15).

"God is a lady", Yusuf told the nurse when he awoke with a quiet smile one Sunday morning. A waxing moon still hung in the sky overhead as the neighbor's rooster spread its tail, calling for all sentient beings to arise. The boy could hear the cook clatter around the kitchen, counting eggs for the boys' breakfasts before church. He suddenly felt as though he was seeing the world for the first time, and he beamed an incandescent smile. His face bore a numinosity the nurse had not seen before, and she stopped what she was doing to stare. "I think God is a woman", Yusuf said, rubbing his eyes, "I feel she likes me. Maybe I am her son".

Never having experienced a mother's love nor a mother's touch, the experience of it in his dreams warmed the child deep down in his soul. He felt himself in a whorl of divine sweetness and had the strange sensation of movement within his bones. "Did you know I am made of water?" he asked the nurse. "It used to be agitated, but the Lady God put my waters calm".

To either psychologist or shaman, his type of numinous, transcendent experience signals a real spontaneous breakthrough, a tangible and naturally occurring phenomenon that could lend itself to guidance in a stable direction, eventually incorporating new cognitions and behaviors. There was a ripe opening for sound theoretical work for the development of character, conscience, responsibility, and healing. This was a benign phenomenon with the potential to soothe and save Yusuf, a transcendent drive full of ripe possibility. In other words, it is a phenomenon that could heal Yusuf rather than one needing healing. According to Ogden (2005), dreaming is the freest, most inclusive and most deeply penetrating form of psychological work of which human beings are capable.

According to Frankl (2000), "What therapy has to achieve is to convert an unconscious *potential* into a conscious *actus* ... to restore it eventually as an unconscious *habitu*s (p. 44). Yusuf expressed a sense of awareness and submission to a force or entity greater than himself, and this was religious regardless of the absence of a specific religious dogma. He spontaneously began to speak the language of his soul in poetry, archetypes, and emotion.

C.G. Jung believed in *anima naturaliter religiosa*, that religiousness is inherent in man, and that even in someone manifestly irreligious, there must be latent religiousness. Other Depth Psychologists believe that religion is only valuable when it is freely chosen rather than driven by an instinct or pushed by culture or creed. Frankl wrote that pressuring someone toward religion along established lines is defeating the purpose.

A ... psychiatrist never has the right to manipulate the patient's Religious feelings by employing religion as just another useful tool to try – along with such things as pills, shots, and shocks. This would be to debase religion and degrade it to a mere device for improving mental health.

(Frankl, 2000, p. 80)

Nevertheless, a naturally occurring religious phenomenon, unbidden by anyone, arose from the boy's unconscious. Whether of a religious nature or simply mythopoetic, Jungian literature is replete with examples of numinous beings and their voices, images, or symbols appearing to people in dreams, visions, speech, and other utterances of the unconscious. These arise from the psyche to help a suffering soul. Psychiatry is advisedly afraid these may amount to commanding voices that urge victims to dark thoughts, including suicide or homicide, but don't forget that such incidents were parred for the course in the ancient world. Remember Francis of Assisi, Hildegard von Bingen, Joan of Arc, and many others.

Hollon and Ferenczi have succinctly explained training for counselors and other mental health practitioners. "The liberation of the mentally ill from the chains of their stigmatization will only become possible if society arrives at an understanding of its madness; if nurses are taught that there is meaning in psychotic talk, and if caregivers analyze their unconscious" (Pestalozzi et al., 1998, as cited in Kafka, 2019).

In traditional cultures, specific training is offered to healers through apprenticeships with shamans. "These societies know (whether) voices stem from evil powers" (Hoffman, 2012). On the other hand, some healers, including some psychiatrists and psychologists, openly disrespect and disavow the potential power of the inner voice for healing, paradoxically expecting voice hearers to turn over such blind-faith authority to themselves instead. This is one of the very reasons for vaccine hesitancy in some cultural contexts during COVID-19. Some articulated, "The world contains so many forms of evil and death. We need a more careful explanation as to which power is presiding now and why we should inject its fluid into our veins".

It is not my intention in this text to discuss therapeutic modalities, but suffice it to say at this juncture that depth psychology provides treatment for the psychoses, which includes the use of mythology, mythopoesis, image, and symbol, even for patients in active psychosis, along with cognitive and behavioral models, and pharmacology, which also have their place.

To complete Yusuf's story, he got out of bed on a cool, grey November morning and began preparing for church. There was new vitality in his movements, new optimism and purposefulness. This perplexed the keeper as she had become accustomed to his normal, which had always been a kind of wispy, rudderless drifting. The keeper now felt disoriented. She decided that the boy would not go to church today. She perceived the dreams he now frequently recounted with stunning clarity as delusional, and she felt there was just too much potential for awkwardness, unpredictability, and disruption. "This boy doesn't know his hand from his foot", she thought. "What then can he know about God?"

She reported the boy's latest conversation to the psychiatrist in charge of the institution, one hierarchical step above the counselor who had thrown in the towel on Yusuf's case sometime before. This one administered the PQ-16, the 16-item version of the Prodromal Questionnaire, to determine the presence and severity of psychosis. The boy scored 12 out of 16 at a level of severe distress. At the same time, the psychiatrist updated his files to include "religious delusion, along with prior manifestations of psychopathy, pedophilia, unexplained somatic complaints and a schizophrenic break with reality". He adjusted the boy's medication to suit, but this psychiatrist had yet to see the boy *qua person.* The doctor more so played the role of voyeur, leaving nothing substantially helpful in his wake. As Fanon often complained, such methodologies myopically reduce the subject to a mere object of examination whereby psychological maladies are dismissed because of a patient's inability to describe them within established and accepted categories.

When the boy aged out of institutional care along with its free health care service, he self-medicated with any street drug he could find.

He overdosed and died one day, never having realized his coming of age as a man. They said his face was peaceful as he went to his grave.

The American Psychological Association reports that death is one outcome of child sexual abuse without explaining just how the road between abuse and death actually unfolds. This, then, is one example.

While Yusuf died young, pursuing any means necessary to achieve that dopamine hit, Carrie lived to old age, never progressing intellectually much past her sensory reactions, forever fearful, suspicious, and on guard.

Fanon and the Child

Franz Fanon (1925–1961) is perhaps best remembered as the first major international psychiatrist to come out of the Caribbean. He is also renowned as an analyst of the gendered and racialized legacies of colonialism, and he has influenced pedagogical, political, and medical practice not only on his island of birth, Martinique but also during his active revolutionary days as a soldier with the Algerian National Liberation Front (1956–1962). A very close reading of Fanon's texts, however, reveals numerous insights into his views on children and childhoods, particularly regarding their upbringing as minority citizens of colonized states, which Bell Hooks named Fanon's "psychopolitics of oppression" (hooks, 2004,). Fanon affords children significant social subjectivity and advocates for a phenomenological approach to attending to them as psychologists. Epistemic primacy should be given to the attitudinal paradigm of the patient's lived experience, he argues, rather than a methodological approach which risks no schematic category existing for that experience.

Where I mention Fanon in this text, I focus on these lesser-known aspects of his legacy, his counter-hegemonic discourse on child raising. He argues that we have come to see our children as colonizers saw and treated us; as ignorant, without self-agency, and in need of strict "spare the rod, spoil the child" control.

His work shows an understanding of the unique competing power relationships between colonizer and colonized, or child and adult, that lends sharp insights into the emotional suffering that may be caused by exploitation, oppression, and alienation. As Burman wrote (2016), this "fruitfully mobilizes other meanings of 'minority' that so materially impact on children as politically disenfranchised based on age and as a minor or subordinated social category" (p. 12).

Writing on Fanon, Burman proposed a unique typology, in much the same vein as Jung, to draw parallels between the psychic violence felt by the disenfranchised, be they colonized nations or colonized nationals. Burman described the metaphorical colonized child as one whose potential for triumphant individuation has been interrupted by the "unnatural" traumatic incident that reverses the developmental path. This interruption renders an entity "already senile before it has come to know the petulance, the fearlessness or the will to succeed of youth" (Fanon, Wretched, p. 123). I feel that this easily applies to the cases presented thus far of Carrie, Melanie, and The Boy. Moreover, as Burman (201) clarified, it is clear that Fanon's primary concern was to understand the impacts of the violence and distortions done to the oppressed/colonized, and to oust these inner psychic reproductions of the colonial state.

Burman's second category in her proposed Fanonian typology of children, is the "gendered and generationally ordered child". Here, Fanon draws linkages between the impacts of colonialism and the anticolonial struggle on inter-generational abuse (Burman, 2016, p. 22). Here, marginalized minorities from the global south have come very far from our Indigenous child-rearing habits, exchanging views of the divine, sacred nature of the child for treatment of them as short, ignorant adults, fully obliged to bear adult indignities of forced labor and forced sex.

In the third and final category, Empirical Children, Burman quotes Fanon, describing "the various assaults made upon them by the very nature of Western culture" (Fanon, EX, pp. 157–158), which includes a purposeful, manufactured vulnerability, suffering, and brutalization. Fanon offers medical case histories as a psychiatrist to illustrate the chronic disturbances caused by the erasure of individual national identity, just as I have offered in this text.

Foster Care, Adoption, and Risk for Sexual Exploitation

Although it is outside the scope of this text to introduce issues of adoption and wider social integration, it must be noted that Yusuf would be extremely difficult to place either within a kinship or foster care setting. Once taken into child protective custody, the process of re-entry into a "natural" family setting becomes fraught. Numerous studies have been conducted on the relationship between children in protective services who have been traumatized and placement stability within new foster settings. Other studies on the relationship between children in protective or foster care and risk factors for sex trafficking and commercial sexual exploitation show youth to be at significant risk for child sexual abuse and commercial sexual victimization, by virtue of being (or having been) within the protective care system in and of itself. In fact, a high-risk youth population is identified as children in foster care.

References

Abramovitch, H., & Kirmayer, L. (2003). The relevance of Jungian psychology for cultural psychiatry. *Transcultural Psychiatry*, *40*(2), 55–163. https://doi.org/10.1177/1363461503402001

Abu-Ras, W., & Abu-Bader, S. J. (2008). The impact of the September 11, 2001, attacks on the well-being of Arab-Americans in New York City. *Journal of Muslim Mental Health*, *3*(2), 217–239. https://doi.org/10.1080/15564900802487634

Alexis, A. (2015). *Fifteen Dogs*. Coach House Press.

Ally, Y., & Laher, S. (2008). South African Muslim faith healers perceptions of mental illness: Understanding, aetiology and treatment. *Journal of Religion and Health*, *47*(1), 45–56. http://www.jstor.org/stable/40344421

American Academy of Family Physicians (2005) www.aafp.org/pubs/afp/issues/2005/0901/p849.pdf

Bailey, M., (2022). *The Art Newspaper*, September 2, 2022. https://www.theartnewspaper.com/2022/09/02. 'My companions in misfortune': discovery reveals who Van Gogh lived with in the asylum (theartnewspaper.com)

Brooks, J. (2015). *Learning from the Lifeworld*. The British Psychological Society. https://www.bps.org.uk/psychologist/learning-lifeworld

Burman, E. (2016). Fanon and the child: Pedagogies of subjectification and transformation. *Curriculum Inquiry*, *46*(3), 265–285. https://doi.org/10.1080/03626784.2016.1168263

Dohe, C. B. (2011). Wotan and the 'archetypal Ergriffenheit': Mystical union, national spiritual rebirth and culture-creating capacity in C. G. Jung's 'Wotan' essay. *History of European Ideas*, *37*(3), 344–356. https://doi.org/10.1016/j.histeuroideas.2010.12.001

Fanon, F. (1967). *The Wretched of the Earth*. Penguin Books.

Fisher, H., Morgan, C., Dazzan, P., Craig, T. K., Morgan, K., Hutchinson, G., Jones, P. B., Doody, G. A., Pariante, C., McGuffin, P., Murray, R. M., Leff, J., & Fearon, P. (2009a). Gender differences in the association between childhood abuse and psychosis. *The British Journal of Psychiatry: the Journal of Mental Science*, *194*(4), 319–325. https://doi.org/10.1192/bjp.bp.107.047985

Frankl, V. (2000) *Man's Search for Ultimate Meaning*, Basic Books.

Goodey, D. (2019). *Frantz Fanon and the Psychology of Oppression: Historical Movements and Movers in Psychology*. Research Gate. https://www.researchgate.net/publication/336878655_Frantz_Fanon_and_the_Psychology_of_Oppression_Historical_Movements_and_Movers_in_Psychology

Gulick, W. B. (1981). Archetypal experiences. *Soundings: An Interdisciplinary Journal*, *64*(3), 237–266. http://www.jstor.org/stable/41178187

Hoffman, M. (2012). *Psychosis as a Personal Crisis: An Experience-Based Approach* (1st ed.). M. Romme & S. Escher (Eds.). Routledge.

hooks, b. (2004). *The Will to Change: Men, Masculinity and Love*. Washington Square Press.

Johnsdotter, S., Ingvarsdotter, K., Östman, M., & Carlbom, A. (2011). Koran reading and negotiation with jinn: Strategies to deal with mental ill health among Swedish Somalis. *Mental Health, Religion & Culture*, *14*(8), 741–755. https://doi.org/10.1080/13674676.2010.521144

Jung, C.G. (1969a) *Collected Works, Vol 9,1. Bollingen Series XX*, Princeton University Press.

Jung, C.G. (1969b) *Collected Works, Vol.8. On the Nature of the Psyche. Translation R.F.C. Hull. Bollingen Series XX*, Princeton University Press.

Jung, C.G. (1973). *Memories, Dreams, Reflections*. Pantheon Books.

Jung, C.G. (1976). *Collected Works, Vol 6 Psychological Types, A Revision by R.F.C. Hull of the Translation by H.G. Baynes*. Princeton University Press.

Kafka, F. (2019). *The Metamorphosis* (I. Johnston, Trans.). *Classics*. (Original work published 1815).

Lorde, A. (2007). *Sister Outsider*. Crossing Press.

Morrison, T. (2017). *The Origin of Others*. Harvard University Press.

Ogden, T. H. (2005). *This Art of Psychoanalysis: Dreaming Undreamt Dreams and Interrupted Cries*. Routledge/Taylor & Francis Group.

Petti, E., Klaunig, M. J., Smith, M. E., Bridgwater, M. A., Roemer, C., Andorko, N. D., Chibani, D., DeLuca, J. S., Pitts, S. C., Schiffman, J., & Rakhshan Rouhakhtar, P. (2023). Mental health care utilization in individuals with high levels of psychosis-like experi-ences: Associations with race and potentially traumatic events. *Cultural Diversity and Ethnic Minority Psychology, 29*(3), 302–315.

Pierre, J. M. (2001). Faith or delusion? At the crossroads of religion and psychosis. *Journal of Psychiatric Practice, 7*(3), 163–172. https://doi.org/10.1097/00131746-200105000-00004

Rahimi, S. (2021). *The Hauntology of Everyday Life.* Palgrave MacMillan.

Rassool, G. H. (2018). *Evil Eye, Jinn Possession, and Mental Health Issues: An Islamic Perspective.* Routledge.

Romme, M., & Escher, S. (Eds.). (2013). *Psychosis as a Personal Crisis: An Experience-Based Approach.* Routledge.

Romme, M., Escher, S., Dillon, J., Corstens, D., & Morris, M. (2013) *Living with Voices: 50 Stories of Recovery.* PCCS Books

Sharp, D. (1987). *Personality Types: Jung's Model of Typology.* Inner City Books.

Sofou, N., Giannakopoulos, O., Arampatzi, E, & Konstantakopoulos, G. (2021). Religious delusions: Definition, diagnosis and clinical implications. *Psychiatrike = Psychiatriki, 32*(3), 224–231. https://doi.org/10.22365/jpsych.2021.014

Von Franz, M., & Hillman, J. (20131). Lectures on *Jung's Typology.* Spring Publications.

Chapter 5

Coco

Coco grew up on the coast of a small fishing village, snuggled into the foothills of a mountain range that stretched upwards and out as far as the eye could see. From the soft ocean at her doorstep, where the lapping of waves and the screaming of gulls were her constant playlist, Coco had only to glance sideways to take in the immensity of the hills at her back, swaddling her in primal green energy. Parrots filled her skies every morning at dawn, flying low enough that the yellow under-sides of their bodies could almost be touched. There was marvel all around her, and nature provided every opportunity for the inhabitants of this idyllic cove to thrive.

Coco's parents were young, educated, ambitious, and hard-working. Both hold-ing corporate jobs during the day and taking professional development courses on-line at night, they were confident in raising a calm, studious, and obedient daughter, the only child they planned to have. When Coco's driver dropped her off after half-day school, a helper waited to let her inside, fix her a snack, and settle her into her homework before knocking off for the day. The rest of the time, before Mum and Dad came in to eat quickly and sit at their laptops, Coco was left to her own devices.

Her "devices" went by the name of Stout, the gardener, her one and only friend until she left home at 15. Stout could be counted upon to run errands on her behalf, to make her dinner if Mr. and Mrs. were late getting home, to climb coconut trees like her personal Spiderman and pull down the sweetest water for her thirst. Stout patched bruised knees, taught her to ride her bicycle, and listened to the stories of her mornings at school. He kept all his promises and was the only one to do that. When he deemed her old enough to handle it, he initiated her into sex. She was about five years old at the time.

> I was invisible to my parents. Not seen, not heard, not engaged in any way for more than about half an hour in the evenings when they got me ready for bed. They shared nothing, showed nothing of themselves, gave me absolutely no sense of who I was or where I belonged in their lives or in this world. I spent hours and hours alone each day. I had mountains of books, but a child can only do so much reading alone. I'm talking years, you know. Years. Thank God for Stout. I was so grateful for his time. The sex fucked me up, pun intended, but

DOI: 10.4324/9781003223603-7

by the pain I knew I was alive. Sex and pain were my only indicators of existence, so I kept going back, not that I had much choice. I wouldn't say he ever
forced me, really; he was just always there. You think I would report him? Or let
anybody find out? I would die first, frankly. What I hated was the slime, though.
There was this constant flow of slime on me. Up to now, if I cough, I feel I'm
bringing up the slime. But anything was better than the black void my parents
left me to exist in. They didn't even brush my hair. I still feel the loneliness. It's
like, cosmic.

As such, Coco did nothing to save herself.

When she was 13, friends of Stout's began to visit in the afternoons. They were
men coming off the sea, traveling through with various forms of cargo, here today,
gone tomorrow. They visited to have sex with Coco, and she soon realized that
Stout was collecting fees and favors for the transactions. At this point, Coco simply
asked him to stop, and he did so with nothing more than a shrug. "Alright", he said,
with his trademark big grin. "Alright, alright, no worries".

Coco walked out of her parent's house at age 15 without a backward glance. She
lied about her age, claiming to be older, and hitched a ride on one of the yachts
at the harbor. She spent the next year jumping from ship to shore, working as a
waitress, bartender, or barrister, or selling herself for money. She actively engaged
in sex with men, women, or trans-people and developed a growing reputation for
aggressive fetishism in the act. By 19, Coco had covered the Mediterranean and
Greek isles, with plans to join a crew headed for New Zealand. Her genes had
gifted her with a body just over six feet tall, highly muscled and toned, the muscle
being all the more articulated by the amount of rope she pulled out at sea.

Inside that body, it was a different story. Coco realized that along with her hyper-
sexuality, she was now becoming aroused by the sexual fear and pain of others. She
would hear or see someone cry, cringe, or experience sexual victimization in some
form, and from out of nowhere, or so she thought, she would become aroused by it.

Coco had grown up surrounded by affluence, and she gravitated to the more
luxurious yachts where even out on the seas, miles from populations, she was still
able to access a bombardment of social media. Sexual images and symbolism came
at her from everywhere, as well as from her own biology. She fought for discern-
ment, integrity, and responsibility, but instead, she found herself washed away by
pungent memories, overwhelmed and disabled.

Coco spiraled down fast, now attempting suicide by diverse creative means. A
deep intrapsychic conflict took root, and caught between an overwhelming desire
to die and an opposite possessing imperative to live, she broke down over and
over again. However, like small trees that fall over when battered by wind and
rain, Coco's roots remained intact, and despite herself, she would spring back. She
began to suspect that an energy more than human within herself was forcing her
to live. Alongside it, equally as powerfully, her nervous system continued to ignite
every time that she heard about or imagined the pain of others, sexual or otherwise.
She finally had to confront the existence of sadistic feelings within herself and the

conflation of sadism with lustful, aggressive fantasies. (This is an example of the especially colorful or intense contents of the "feeling-toned" complexes to which Jung refers.)

Repulsed by the thoughts in her mind and exhausted by the mental effort it took to keep them at bay, Coco felt fatigued around the clock. No matter how much she slept, she woke up tired, but although she kept refining her commitment to suicide, something in her refused to die. Finally, when she witnessed an adolescent girl dragged below deck by a sex tourist and experienced an almost visible, full-blown thrill, Coco knew it had gone too far. She felt like two separate people, herself and then her body existing alongside herself with a brain and sensations of its own. Coco felt driven to outrun this auxiliary body, and this accounted for her extreme adventures at sea, deep free-diving, para-gliding in storm-strength gales, and fishing with spear guns. Alternatively, she would shut down completely via designer drugs, prescription drugs, or full depressive collapse.

At about this time, Coco lost another personal, intimate relationship. Her current boyfriend became afraid rather than thrilled by her cold, dominatrix persona, and she knew it was time to take a pause, catch her breath, and face the demons festering inside. With a new stable land job as a waitress in a restaurant overlooking a tiny cove much like the one she'd grown in, Coco paused just long enough to let herself break down. Triggered by nothing she could recall, she began to shake, sweat, weep, and call out to no one there. When she fell to the floor in unconscious convulsions, an ambulance was called, which took her to the nearest psychiatric institution. Coco was treated with enough anti-psychotic medication to fell a racehorse and to keep her down again every time her consciousness began to stir.

Coco had also experienced a bout of psychogenic non-epileptic seizures, as described in the previous chapter on Yusuf, but once again, psychiatric staff neither explored this diagnosis nor any that connected Coco's seizures to child abuse psychosis.

When she was released a week later, and the same ugly emotions surfaced to molest her some more, Coco made a conscious decision to institutionalize herself for a longer term, where drugs would take her completely out of herself. Where some victims of child trauma describe blankness, memory loss, and dissociation, Coco's memories only sharpened with time and consumed her, leaving her powerless in their grip, dominated, or possessed. "Something is taking me", she often said, and it was many years before she could articulate much more than that to a therapist. As Dieckmann wrote, "It is difficult to clinically reconstruct the elements of very early personal experience since they lie outside the realm of voluntary recall in the earliest periods of life" (Dieckmann, 1999, p. 45).

Nevertheless, at this point in her breakdown, Coco craved and benefitted from psychiatry's traditional capacity for playing a medication-only role, especially sedation.

She made her voluntary return to the institution late one evening. In the parking lot of that hospital, Coco stretched out her physique, all six foot, 200 pounds of her, and loosened her hair to stand up straight in all directions like the Statue of Liberty.

She pranced and hollered from the depths of her soul, "Watch me! I'm going mad! I'm going mad here now!"

The only entity at the institution with any capacity for handling Coco was the head nurse, a woman of equal physical size and strength with absolutely no compassion.

"None of your shit", she told Coco, "None of that shit here". Beckoning the orderlies, she saw about restraining, subduing, and administering enough neuroleptic (anti-psychotic) medication to displace all positive symptoms of the psychosis, along with any possibility of resistance, thereby restoring peace and order to her ward and dispatching Coco to that spectral space of haunted nonbeing that she had come for; that she craved and had called to herself; a virtual exorcism of the agony in her soul. Through a Martin-Baro lens, the head nurse's psychology describes a philosophy of practice that exists to serve the institution's interests rather than the patient. One far-reaching consequence of this is that if none of a mental health patient's life stories are heard, along with the social, historical, and biological genesis of their diseases, then no effective *preventive* measure will ever be conceived and implemented in order to forestall them. Moreover, reading this point of view with Paolo Freire, we can also see his notion of *conscientization* brought into the service of a *system* rather than of a people as he intended.

As Coco claimed her "right to sickness", weariness descended upon her like molten lead, and she only wanted to sleep for a very long time. Human rights always include the freedom to say no to freedom, and Coco exercised that right, willingly surrendering herself to be caged. She was officially diagnosed with schizophrenia with extremely violent tendencies and a high potential for dangerousness both to herself and others. Over the course of the next three years, Coco volunteered herself for confinement five times. At no point in that time did she ever have in-depth conversations with the psychiatrist or other staff, nor did they show much interest in getting to know her. The intimacy of scrutiny would have been too much to bear (for either Coco or her helpers). In Coco's case, drugs were her much-preferred option over facing the unbearable realities of her past and present life.

As Douglas Noble wrote in 1963, describing a mental health facility in the USA, "Underlying the therapeutic program was the theory that the schizophrenic patient, because of early hurts to his ego, required a long period of affectionate care in which his trust in another person would be restored and intensive therapeutic work would then be possible." However, moving all the way forward to 2019, such necessary professionals were still the exception, by far, rather than the rule.

> One doctor ... was remarkably successful in treating extremely traumatized patients, conveyed to us his therapeutic strategy of spending much time with his patients exploring every detail of their positive, not traumatic, memories.
>
> (Kafka, 2019, p. 111)

Additionally, in confirmation of the truth that inadequate therapeutic care for victims of child abuse psychosis is not only an issue for developing but for developed countries as well, Mark Blechner reflects on his psychiatric work at a New York psychiatric institute, writing that "The ability to communicate with anyone, especially with psychotics, is a skill that I think is gradually being lost today in mainstream psychiatry" (Blechner, 2019, p. 111)

Coco and the Nurse were different sides of one coin. Coco was determined to suppress her troubling thoughts through self-harming compulsions, and Nurse was determined to subdue others by submission and the removal of their freedoms.

> An unconscious drama is then played out in which the helper, clothed in the persona of selfless concern, unconsciously asserts her will over the client. At the other pole of the interchange sits the client, clothed in a compliant persona while unconsciously resisting the helper's domination and belittlement.
>
> (Guggenbuhl-Craig, 2015, p. 15)

Patriarchal systems are always hierarchical, with those who feel themselves to be without power having no greater dream than to rise to power, not in terms of self-agency, but in terms of power over others.

As another resident of a different institution wrote:

> In the mental hospital, I was locked like an animal in a cage; no one came when I called, begging to be taken to the bathroom, and I finally had to succumb to the inevitable. Blessedly, I was given daily shock treatment, insulin shock, and sufficient drugs so that I lost most of the next several weeks …
>
> (Frankl, 2000)

In many parts of the world, stigma and discrimination against mental illness, considering both label avoidance and public stigma, prevent many from seeking help for their painful feelings. Job offers, the social standing of entire kinship networks, and even anticipated proposals of marriage could be put in jeopardy based on rumors of poor mental health in one family member. However, Coco had long ago ceased to care what any public thought of her. In fact, considering the social circles in which she normally moved, if Coco mentioned to anyone that she had been institutionalized several times for "madness", they found her heroic and all the more alluring.

In one of her last gigs as a yachting crew, before Coco left the scene to attend to her health, she found work on board a luxury craft where a young girl child was among the group. Coco saw herself in the child and began to court a friendship with her. The family was only too happy to have the child tended so enthusiastically by a female helper, leaving her to Coco's devices more and more. The child was pure innocence and joy, and at first, Coco followed her around, watching her play, simply to remind herself what inherent innocence was like. She captured the images in photographs, and in the evenings, Coco scrolled her smartphone galleries scrutinizing the happy faces, the surprised expressions, the little girl's tantrums, and tears. She felt herself heavily identified with the child and even began to learn from her, particularly in the realm of her open-armed embrace of affection and her ability to rebound so quickly from tears, spills, and fears. If the child tripped over something and fell, burned her fingers on a stove, or drew back confused from chastising words, Coco held her tight and comforted her, absorbing the surges of all the various emotions running through the little body.

Inexplicably, Coco was fired one day. She was given no warning, no notice, no severance pay. A dinghy simply pulled up alongside the yacht in the middle of a calm, blue sea, and she was instructed to get on. "You need to be grateful we don't put you in jail, you sick fuck!" Coco had no idea what she had done to merit this but sought relief in the one familiar thing that she knew: pain. Burning herself with fire from a match was now her preferred method of self-harming, but she had developed an arsenal of choices over the years.

It is crucial to note that while Coco had recognized and been horrified by the sadistic tendencies arising in herself sometime before, she drew no parallels between those and the harmful behaviors she had engaged with the child. She had cultivated a loving, trusting relationship with the girl and believed that all of her choices in her regard were pure, despite the fact that she had well crossed those boundaries by the time she was discovered. "I am innocent", she kept repeating years after the incidents. To date, she has never allowed herself to contemplate anything other than the purest motives coming from herself to "her" child. Even if the law had taken Coco into custody and charged her with child abuse, she would never accept culpability. To press this point further, even if Coco had been forced to articulate a confession of abuse for any legal reason, psychologically speaking, she would never have believed her own words. She was holding out for the innocence of her own inner child, holding on by the molars, a virtual matter of life or death for her own soul.

By age 25, it was fair to say that Coco found herself fully broken, though she continued to find work, socialize, post gorgeous photographs to media, laugh out loud, and live a life that many envied.

In psychotherapy with Coco, I needed to move like a hunter in a forest, treading gently, minding my breath, and calculating my words. On the one hand, I needed a straightforward cognitive-behavioral strategy for managing her emotions, thoughts, and lifestyle choices so that she could continue to make a living and function in the world. On another level, I worked in collaboration with a psychiatrist to provide, monitor, and adjust the medications that helped keep her stable. Additionally, a psychosocial responsibility was to have her agree to keep away from under-aged children while we completed psychological work. But at root, only a Depth Psychological approach could help Coco rid herself of the sense of personal badness that she had carried all of her life and was now so deeply embedded in her psyche that she could no longer uncover where it lay, except that it "possessed" her and continued to inform all of her adult choices. For Coco to confront that she had finally become what she most despised, an abuser of small children without guilt, remorse, or even acknowledgment of the fact, would cause her to see herself as beyond any redemption, and that would certainly give her the wherewithal to complete her suicide ideation once and for all.

Considering Carl Rogers' version of the hypocritic oath, in which you do not engage a client unless you can guarantee your capacity to give them "unconditional positive regard", it is fair to say that psychotherapy is not for the faint of heart. When facing such clients as Coco, the sheer velocity of her psychic weight alone, never mind the plethora of psychosocial and interpersonal issues, leaves the best practitioners shivering in their shoes.

For me personally, after so many years in this work where darkness lurks in all corners, I find myself reaching increasingly for a deeper knowledge of the neuroscience of trauma and equally for a deepening appreciation of the psychology of religion. I feel no conflict in this approach, but that is an exploration for a subsequent text.

Another client described her gradual descent into child abuse psychosis in these words.

Doctor, is it possible for me to fall down, shaking up and bawling because of sex? I started with sex when I was very young, maybe ten years old or so. My mother let men touch me. She ran a bar and grocery as her source of income, so when I came home from school, I stayed in the back room doing homework. Men came in the back and groped me, and squeezed my breasts. I told my Mum. She replied, "Oh God, you want to kill me?" I was so very astonished by her response and so confused by it I didn't know what to say, so I never brought it up again. When the men started raping me on the flour sacks, I just let it happen. I cried for my mother, but I cried silently not to bother her.

Later on, I passed my college exams and went to board with an auntie in town. It was a good place, and she was a real mother to me. When I graduated college, I had high marks and got a good job at a bank. I was so happy. I had saved myself. Now, to find my own apartment, I found the bank salary could not really stretch to reach a cost of living. A couple of colleagues, male as well as female, told me about the escort business with tourist people. It made good money. Real money. And no problem for me as I grew up like that. Nobody in society knew. We were a hidden population. I don't have more to say about that, but I could finally earn a living.

Then I met my husband and he was a really good man. We got married; who would believe that? He treats me like a queen. But he has a really high sex drive, and sometimes, in the middle of it, just when one part of me actually starts to relax, let go, and take pleasure in this, another voice in my head shouts out, "No! No! Don't let go! Grip! Grip!" Then I get all tensed up and that is when I start shaking and heaving and bawling out. If I get up, I fall down. I roll on the ground. The voices take over, telling me, "Grip! Grip!".

My poor husband. He cries. Some people tell him I have schizophrenia and other people tell him that somebody "do" me so I am going between the psychiatrist and the pastor. Now I'm asking you, doctor, can this kind of a breaking down come from sex?

A Fanonian View of the Colonized States
of Individual Mind

Thinking this through with Fanon, so to speak, he saw the colonial world as divided into ordered but conflicting compartments. In Wretched of the Earth, he was writing about the Algerian National Liberation Front in the 1950s but his concepts can also easily be applied to the war that is raging between the Palestinian people and the settler colonial state of Israel, even as I write these words. In either case, the compartmentalization of conflicting parts also applies to the fractured psyche of the victimized and oppressed individual, as in the case of the abused child.

In the case of the state, Fanon describes frontiers bordered by barracks, police stations, and soldiers, and a middle ground that contains moral guardians who hand out rewards for submission and good behavior. He refers to a multitude of moral teachers, counselors, and bewilders who separate the exploited from those in power while themselves ensuring that the violence of oppression remains intact, though muted and disguised. Similarly, this prostituted client's psyche was colonized and occupied by the number of men who abused her at the frontier and then by her employers, the gatekeepers in the middle ground, who provided such low salaries that the client was kept submissive and beholden to various colonizing or patriarchal authorities. Finally, there is the conflict set up by the psyche's super-ego, rushing forward as it is wont to do to save a person's soul by flooding them with guilt in the form of the call "Grip, grip". This is the wisdom of the guilt complex, cautioning against daring to enjoy the very activity that was once used to enslave it. These conflicting forces, Fanon suggests, are not rational but emanate from a dualistic Manichean world, which exerts a great force throughout. To oppress a child is to disfigure and deform its beauty, Fanon writes, rendering the child a depository of "maleficent power" (Fanon, p. 32).

Depth psychology's therapeutic modality called "Parts Work" was specifically developed as an intervention that helps us understand the unique layout of our internal landscapes, integrating and restabilizing the many fractured parts of a pathologized psyche.

In Ana Mozol's 2019 text, A Re-Visioning of Love: Dark Feminine Rising, she writes:

> It is certain that life is never the same and that one does not return to one's previous state of being. A woman who has touched this abyss through violation knows in the cells of her being the futility of most living: she can't engage in the pleasantries of being proper and alive – although she may try. The demon takes up primary residence in her dreams, night terrors, sexual fantasies, bodily symptoms (panic attacks, vaginismus, infections, indiscriminate pain, migraines), and psychotic attachments (repetitive abusive relationships). It does not let go, not without hard and painful work. I would venture to say many women suffering from such a complex remain unaware that their lives are controlled by an inner demon unless, by grace, they are offered the opportunity to

feel safe enough to unravel, reveal, and explore the intolerable image. In fact, in analysis, it may take years for the dreams and fantasies confirming this state of possession to surface or for a woman to risk sharing them. Initially, there is often an enormous degree of shame surrounding them.

(Mozol, 2019, p. 29)

Artemis: Archetypal Energy in the Helping Professions

In my childhood, I ran on naked feet through the properties my parents and their extended families and friends owned or visited, feeling a deep affinity with nature, the earth, and her surrounding seas. Each morning, I awoke to my mother's meditation: "I lift mine eyes onto the hills from whence cometh my strength," and in the evenings, I listened to stories of my father's hunt through the woods of St. David's, nothing to slow him down but his companions. Sundays were days for fishing off the Quarantine Station point or along the Eastern coastline in Belle Isle, where I learned patience, silent abiding, and how to watch the waters for movement. I never received better training for psychotherapeutic work than this. Wait, watch, and stay alert. Don't judge. Phenomena are perpetually arising.

In mythology, Artemis is the Greek Goddess of the hunt and the moon. She roams the wilderness, armed with a bow and quiver of arrows, the protector of girls and small animals. She has an indomitable spirit and cannot be subdued. Additionally, Artemis is associated with mystical and meditative experiences, a sensing of subtle energies, and a capacity for inner reflection.

In Jungian psychology, the eight major goddesses defined in classical mythology represent archetypal patterns and energies that are active in every person, a part of the innate natural gifts and personalities with which each of us comes to the world. These gifts will either be recognized and supported by our parents and carers or beaten out of us, depending on the families we have and the social expectations of the day. Child sexual abuse has the directed purpose of annihilating the goddess in girls (or the gods in boys). However, an a priori essence remains, perhaps lying dormant until it is safe to raise its head or until a torch is extended to light the way out of darkness.

Many women who…came from families where parental figures neglected, rejected, or abused them emotionally or physically…find solace in nature or with animals… nature provides animals with protective coloring so they don't stand out. When animals are wounded or weakened, they know how to hide their vulnerability to avoid becoming prey.

(Bolen, 2014, p. 18)

Mythology is a wonderful vehicle via which Jungian psychologists gather stories, images, feelings, and depth that illustrate experiences and characters we can identify with. Where insights lead us to recognize aspects of ourselves that we did not realize before, an archetypal energy is ushered into life that can be meaningful and powerfully liberating. (Jean Shinoda Bolen, 2014). Not only a popular figure in works of art over the centuries, Artemis shows up in contemporary fiction and film (Bobby & Harney, 2016), such as the character Katniss Everdeen in Suzanne Collin's *The Hunger Games* (2008), in Rick Riordan's *Percy Jackson and the Olympians* book series and the 1990s TV series *Hercules: The Legendary Journeys*. Also a symbol of swiftness and accuracy, Artemis was invoked by the professional yacht racing team *Artemis Racing*, which I was thrilled to watch train for the America's Cup when I visited my daughter and her family in Bermuda in 2016. In 2022, NASA launched a complex mission to enable humans to explore the Moon and Mars, Artemis I, with Artemis II scheduled to launch in 2024. Artemis III, holding to its mythological origins, will be the first craft to carry female, black astronauts into space sometime after 2024. Artemis is also embodied in individual women; Gloria Steinem, Jane Goodall, Alice Walker, Mia Motley, and Malala Yousafzai are just some.

Most poignantly for me, however, Artemis is an archetypal ideal of feminism, activism, and psychotherapy.

> Whether or not women know it, Artemis is the archetype or goddess who can inspire us to be activists in the world.
>
> (Gloria Steinem, quoted in Bolen, 2014)

According to C.G. Jung, archetypes come out of the collective unconscious, which is shared by all human beings, unlike the personal unconscious. They represent images, feelings, and behaviors that have existed since we can remember ; however, "the archetype always meets the need of the moment" (CW, vol. 5ii, p. 450).

While psychiatrists and MDs looked for the diagnostic sources of Coco's epileptic episodes, various gastrointestinal problems, and immune system malfunctions, in terms of biology, they did not extend themselves to the psychosomatic, nor even to the plain psycho. Coco became a docile recipient of care, an isolated, controllable invalid, just as she'd been conditioned to be.

Very few people, about 3%, or 3 in 100, will experience an episode of psychosis in their lifetime. Schizophrenia is one of the more serious psychotic disorders, but only about 1% of people will develop it in a lifetime (Compton & Broussard, 2009). Yet, in some parts of the world, it is reported that a much higher percentage of mentally ill people are schizophrenic. If this statistic is true, we urgently need new research to establish linkages in cultures where both sexual violence and psychosis or schizophrenia are similarly high.

References

Blechner, M. (2019). Aspects of clinical work with psychotic patients. In R. Lombardi, L. Rinaldi, & S. Thanopoulos (Eds.), *Psychoanalysis of the Psychoses* (pp. 107–119). Routledge.

Bobby, S., & Harney, E. (Eds.) (2016). *The Artemis Archetype in Popular Culture: Essays on Fiction, Film and Television*. McFarland & Company, Inc.

Bolen, J. S. (2014). *Artemis: The Indomitable Spirit in Everywoman*. Conari Press.

Compton, M., & Broussard, B. (2009). *The First Episode of Psychosis: A Guide for Patients and Their Families*. Oxford University Press.

Dieckmann, H. (1999). *Complexes: Diagnosis and Therapy in Analytical Psychology.* Chiron Publishers.

Frankl, V. (2000). *Man's Search for Ultimate Meaning*. Perseus Publishing.

Guggenbuhl-Craig, A. (2015). *Power in the Helping Professions.* Spring Publications.

Kafka, F. (2019). *The Metamorphosis* (I. Johnston, Trans.). *Classics*. (Original work published 1815).

Mozol, A. (2019). *A Re-Visioning of Love: Dark Feminine Rising* (1st ed.). Routledge.

Chapter 6

Nile

Nile was six years old when his family began to make remarks about him being womanish. He lived in a humble home at the edge of the city with his parents and siblings, who practiced a fundamentalist religion. By age seven, when they deemed he had been "formed", they told him that his effeminate mannerisms risked infecting the whole family, so they sent him to sleep underneath the house at night. Nile was allowed no bedding for the dirt floor, but in the mornings, he was let into the house to wash before school to keep a clean image. His father began a series of ritualized beatings at the same time, and by age eight, Nile began to contemplate suicide. At ten, when the beating rituals escalated in intensity and with which no one interfered, Nile left home, never to return. He set off into the forest one night, looking for somewhere else to be, someone else to become.

In tropical rain forests at night, nature comes alive with snarls, howls, and long, dry tendrils dragging at your cheeks. In Nile's country, where approximately 85% of its 53,104,435 acres is covered by forest, there are over 1300 known species of birds and mammals (and amphibians), and some of them like to get about at night. The thick undergrowth, dense with pungent and rotting foliage, clings to your feet as you walk, making the going perilous and slow. Even in the light of day, the sun's rays are often hard-pressed to shine through. At night, the dank and musty woodlands feed the active imaginations of travelers with images of ghouls and thieves, of ancestors arguing with the gods over the fate of a loved one, of underworld creatures scheming to eat a child, of dead souls stalking. The fragrance of the night is hallucinatory, the taste of the atmosphere salty with fear. Hardly a comforting place for the most adult among us, it is a haunted house for a young boy. But Nile took a belly-deep breath and pressed on. Nothing ahead could be worse than where he had been. He intended life to change.

Von Franz (1990) wrote of the primeval forest as a location for the psychological dark night of the soul or journey of individuation. Hillman similarly described these quests as a "soul-making vale", the destiny factor in everyone's life, shaping our intentions and guiding us. Numerous fairy tales also use the forest as a metaphor for neglected children's salvation, including Goldilocks, Red Riding Hood, and Hansel and Gretel, to name just a few. In West African literature, the Dahomey people tell of the Aziza Faerie, tiny people of the forest who live among ant hills

DOI: 10.4324/9781003223603-8

and silk cotton trees, have magical powers, and help travelers survive the most wicked of circumstances. In the case of Nile, as he quaked in his boots yet pressed on through his very real soul's quest, he felt determined to survive by any means at all. He heard his own teeth rattle with fear, and his psychic pain was real, but inside himself, he bore the *Coeur du lion*, and he moved steadfastly on.

By daybreak, Nile came upon an abandoned farmer's shack, and he went in, remaining there for the next eight years. He found that he had located himself about a mile from one of the country's hinterland tribes, and although they gave each other a wide berth, he sometimes found some smoked meat left just inside his door, and once he found a pan, matches, a sharp blade, and a fishing pole. Thus, given the tools of survival, Nile foraged enough fruit and vegetables to eat, learned to fish, and eventually began to plant not only vegetables but the flowers that caught his eyes purely for their beauty.

Against all odds, Nile was finally able to sustainably harvest enough produce to take into town to sell, and he began asking for odd jobs as a gardener. The gods had gifted this child with a natural affinity for tending plants, and as he pushed through adolescence, he developed a reputation as an intuitive and sensitive landscaper. Everything that he touched blossomed. "Your hands are blessed", people told him. He was hired to do steady work for a large hotel, along with several smaller residences, but at the end of the day, Nile invariably returned to his home at the edge of the forest, as Rainer Maria Rilke might say, to a house beyond all that is far.

At age 25, however, Nile still carried the suicidal ideations that had surfaced in him when he was eight. He told his therapist that, in fact, although he had certainly achieved a good measure of success literally by his own two hands, he increasingly felt that real success would be to pass quietly into the hereafter. He had success, but he had no joy. "If I kill myself now and they find me swinging, they will say that I was a successful man with many colleagues in my business, and they will wonder what happened overnight, but this is not overnight. This is a quarter of a century at least. No one takes the time to listen to my tale."

Psychological Services in Small, Resource-Strapped Communities: A Case Study

The Non-Governmental Organization (NGO) representing the LGBTQI+ community in the town closest to Nile's hotel hosted social events from time to time. For many of the Gay population in the unrelentingly homophobic place that small communities can be, they only socialized in private clubs and agencies for fear of active discrimination from those outside of their group. At those events, Nile said, "I had sex with everybody. Anybody I could get. Condoms were the last thing on my mind." But he added, "I just feel so lonely. I actually do not want this. All I want is one faithful and truly caring person of my own, somebody to belong to."

Most psychological issues surfacing in the LGBTQI+ communities of traditional cultures over the last two or three decades have centered on counseling around HIV/AIDS. In the Caribbean, the second most-affected region in the worldafter

Africa, the Global Fund, the World Bank, and other international agencies have poured billions of dollars into the region for stemming the tide. In 2017 alone, $315 million U.S. was made available. In 2019, 330,000 people were living with HIV (Avert, 2019) but deaths by HIV-related illnesses have now declined by 23%.

Stigma and Discrimination, bullying, family and relationship breakdown, and physical violence, including suicide and murder, are common for this population. According to the Observatory of Murdered Trans People, between 25 and 30 transgender people have been murdered each year between 2008 and 2020, 78% of them coming from Latin America and the Caribbean (Avert, 2019). The psychological traumas associated with these facts are significant. White et al. (2010) name "minority stress," major depression, generalized anxiety disorder, conduct disorder, and nicotine dependence, as well as school-related dysfunction in the youth demographic (Bagley & D'Augelli, 2000; De Graaf et al., 2006). Furthermore, it has been established that poor relationships within low-income families such as Nile's, within the discriminated LGBTQI population are predictive of poor mental health outcomes throughout the lifespan.

However, most psychosocial services offered to this population have traditionally focused on VCT (Voluntary Counseling and Testing), along with advanced medical treatments. The primary intention has been to solve medical emergencies, with socio-political issues coming next and depth psychology either lagging well behind or being non-existent.

Nearly, 70% of participants in this demographic met the criteria for an Axis I disorder in their lifetime, but only about 10% reported ever receiving counseling. In most communities, the mental health needs of sexual minorities remain largely unmet. Improving the human resource capacity of local human rights and LGBTQI+ support groups to offer interventions by trained mental health professionals, as well as ensuring that public health facilities are better responsive to these needs, is also essential in reducing mental health risks among sexual minorities.

Nile regularly attended VCT sites for testing, normally within the week following a social event when he was racked with fear, guilt, shame, and various other deeply troubling feelings. Along with testing his HIV status, he always requested psychological counseling, naming his presenting issue as: "I have a pain in my soul". The first three psychologists from whom Nile sought relief for his soul suffering are representative of numerous similar reports, not only across the Latin and Caribbean region, but throughout the wider world.

Psychologist One belonged to an NGO that received a grant to address the HIV epidemic through education and condom distribution. This was their primary mechanism for preventing HIV transmission. The Psychologist needed to submit reports to his donors that quantified his results, or he would lose his financing and, thus, his livelihood. He gave Nile some tracks, pamphlets, and free condoms and sternly reprimanded him to "wrap it up!"

"Never mind your loneliness," he said. "You make that condom your best friend! Just wrap it up!" Nile's bid for conversations that probed the meaning of self and his ongoing search for his lost soul was inconvenient to that counselor, who moved quickly through his checklist and on to the next in line. It bodes mentioning that many state-insurance-run healthcare systems in first-world cities operate in the same way. Many counseling services reflect strapped resources where contact is made, and documentation is taken, but no substantive psychological help is offered. Unfortunately, in times of restriction and contraction in the global south, this becomes more of the rule than the exception, and there are no regulatory bodies to provide supervision.

Psychologist Two, in Nile's case, had a law degree as well as psychological credentials. He explained to Nile that he was suffering from Christian guilt about his sexual activity but had the fundamental human right to have sex with as many partners as he wanted to. Nile got a human rights lecture and was reminded that because of the success of the black power and feminist movements, gay rights were now also internationally upheld (except in the reality of many traditional cultures), so Nile was actually living in a good time, standing on the shoulders of the mighty. Nile's articulated desire to settle into one committed relationship was treated with disdain, as though infantile, and he was reminded once again that he was privy to an enviable freedom of attractive choice.

Writing of much more than just race, Toni Morrison (2017) said, "For humans as an advanced species, our tendency to separate and judge those not in our clan as the enemy, the vulnerable and the deficient needing control, has a long history" (p. 3). Similarly, Jungian psychology is always looking for the prejudices that various collectives carry, in which certain behaviors and habits are discouraged; "Never in our family", we may say. Or, "We just don't do that here!" The LGBTQI+ community, along with almost all other communities seeking political and social cohesion, often demands "at oneness" from its members, but little do we expect a barrier to the process of individuation to come from within the psychological community itself. Nevertheless, in clinical practice as in communities, there is no wonder that the earlier, all-powerful collective persona prevented objective psychological evaluation of individual differences or individual psychological processes. Brooke writes that the development of identity, or the process of individuation, is always, to some degree, a compromise with the larger collective. He says, "This amounts to submersion in the anonymity of the collective life where 'they' become a new kind of Mother, and true individuality and consciousness, which is founded on dialogue with the self, is lost" (Brooks, 2015, p. 23).

Frankl wrote that hyper-intention is often behind the mass emphasis on sexual achievement. He believed that a will to sexual pleasure and happiness is, in fact, a frustrated will to *meaning*. "Sexual libido only hypertrophies in an existential vacuum. The result is an inflation of sex … associated with a devaluation" (Frankl, 2000, p. 90).

I am by no means prepared to argue that this is always the case. The sexual liberation movement, which blossomed in the sixties as a result of cultural transformations, medical and scientific discoveries, and feminism, put an end to sexual repression and oppression and allowed a diversity of sexual identities and practices to come to light. Importantly, it also drove legal reform and human rights amendments for non-heteronormative populations, allowing us to move sex out of a purely reproductive or conjugal framework. But in the case of this client, Nile, as is the case with many clients, regardless of gender or cultural affiliation, his unique psychological crisis was subverted to the interests of other motives. As such, his sexual neurosis was as much a para-clinical or sociogenic neurosis as it was personal.

Psychotherapy needs to keep conscious of moving away from its own reductionism to consistently refresh and rehumanize itself, lest we find ourselves reinforcing rather than counteracting our clients' and cultures' ills. However, empiricism often fails to open itself to the realm of the meanings in language, sticking to what seems purely factual in the view of each individual practitioner. With populations as diverse as ours, speaking globally as well as in the context of Latin America and the Caribbean, there is no way to homogenize the way we go mad nor is it possible to homogenize treatments.

As opposed to the first psychologist, who was simply more interested in the administration of his NGO than his individual clientele, the second is an example of projective identification, in which the therapist took it for granted that his client had the same feelings as himself and advised him in accordance with that assumption. Here, therapist number two likely wanted to rid *himself* of Christian guilt for any number of reasons, and lobbed that projection toward his client, not only assuming but indicating that he should feel the same way. Though Nile asserted "But I'm sick. I feel emotionally sick. I need help and you're not hearing me," Psychologist Two persisted in advising him to free himself from the shackles of mental slavery. Neither heard nor understood, Nile was left to unravel some more.

Number Three was a psychologist who also carried the title "Patient Advocate" and was a PLWA (Person living with AIDS). He had been trained in New York and set out to inject positivism and confidence into his client's life. He disclosed that he had suffered similar torments as Nile, isolated himself for long periods of time, and contemplated suicide. Now, he embraced his hypersexual lifestyle and sincerely wanted Nile to do the same, in accordance with his own "true" nature.

This was another projection where the therapist identified with the client's background so thoroughly that he unconsciously merged himself with the client, ignoring Nile's individual process, and coercing Nile to act and feel as he, the therapist, did. Nile's ongoing quest for saving his own mortal soul; a process which began so long ago in his family of origin, now found itself once again thwarted by his projectively-identifying psychotherapist. This is another example of individuality being suppressed, perhaps inadvertently, in favor of the overwhelming force of the collective group mind or participation mystique.

According to Jung, when the personality overly attempts to adapt to the collective, losing touch with the self, sickness of the soul arrives. This applies to members of any marginalized community who feel oppressed by the dominant order as well as by mainstream psychology. Freud also commented that ties of identification connect mankind in various directions and to numerous social networks, and while this may be normal and good, it also exposes us to all the group psyches that emanate from each person's race, class, and nationality. Individuals are often hard pressed to rise above all of this collective energy, unless powerfully motivated to remain independent and unique. In *The Undiscovered Self*, Jung wrote that the doctor (therapist) is faced with the task of treating a person with psychic suffering, with individual understanding. We need to look at concrete individuals, not mass formations and not organizations. Although anxiety leads us to search for the familiar and comfortable inexperience and to throw out the rest, therapists who merge with psychological mass-mindedness lose their professional dignity as well.

Participation Mystique

Participation Mystique is a theoretical idea first proposed by anthropologist Levy-Bruhl and later taken up by Jung, which describes that if we go all the way back to the first or indigenous psychologies, there is no trace of the individuation aims currently espoused by Depth Psychology. Rather, as Jung wrote, "most connections in the world are not relationships, they are participation mystique. One is then apparently connected, but of course it is never a real connection, it is never a relationship, but it gives the feeling of being one sheep in the flock at least" (Jung. Visions. P. 625). In Jung's theory of the five stages of consciousness, participation mystique is the lowest stage (Stein, 1998, p. 179).

I take this as an expansion of the framework of bystander mobilization, which considers the principles of participation mystique as central. Fanny Brewster brings the collectivist cultural concept of Africanism to the table. She says, "The philosophical underpinnings of many African traditions and social systems are that the collective is of primary importance. It is of greater importance than the individual" (Brewster, 2020, p. 62).

While this is certainly true of collective societies, we need to be on the lookout for where this very tenet may be brought into the service of evil, as the normalization of child sexual abuse and its attendant silencing for the sake of the family, may be taken as an utter betrayal of both individualist *and* collectivist cultures. It is rather in the very strength of a fully individuated person that their capacity for meaningful contribution to the collective lies. In my experience as a clinician working with an extremely diverse clientele, I have seen collectivism privileged over individualism, where CSA exists in families who would do anything rather than speak out against the significant harm being done to the children in their midst.

When Nile began psychological work with me, he presented with a list of compelling issues, including child abandonment, neglect, physical, sexual and spiritual abuse, and sexually aggressive, predatory behaviors of his own. He described mourning the loss of his parents and home, of his youth and all that was familiar. Nile also retained an inherent drive to be independent and original, and in the meanwhile, he sought determinedly to fill the empty void with endless sexual couplings, which left him empty inside, melancholic, and increasingly suicidal. He was now actively placing himself at medical risk, and actively exposing others to risk of infection as well. None of this had been addressed by any of the three attending psychologists he described and clearly this is dangerously problematic. What is called for, from a phenomenological point of view, is to leave reductionist indoctrination behind, along with any pre-conceived patterns of interpretation and simply turn to the heart of the man, or to the wisdom of the heart. We must listen deeply before we venture to respond.

Hans Strupp, a pioneer in the empirical study of brief psychodynamic therapy and one of the founders of the field of psychotherapy research, left us with a number of rich studies of the interplay of hostility between client and therapist. He found evidence that even very subtle negative or blaming comments on the part of the therapist appeared to have a negative impact on the outcome of psychotherapy. These were typically comments that could be seen as both supportive and somewhat blaming. Strupp's work adds empirical weight to the theoretical insights of writers such as Meares and Hobson, Wile, and Wachtel, who cautioned against what might be called the "pejorative tendency" in psychological practice.

It is not the behavior-change psychological modalities that have theory and skills for getting to the depths of the soul traumas that plague multitudes of individuals like Nile in vulnerable communities the world over. It is a Depth perspective that is called for, and we have already seen it successfully applied and embedded within the Latin American and Eurocentric Caribbean, where psychological themes are not dissimilar. The Black Caribbean, however, has been summarily left out. However, not only is a psychoanalytic or Depth psychological approach urgent for this demographic, but almost more importantly so for their psychologists, who face rolling tides of global inequities, injustices, abuses, and the ongoing, escalating maltreatment of children and the vulnerable, yet are not always educated in the full array of tools and technologies for assisting their clientele.

Most Caribbeans have retained strong though silent ties to their ancestral belief systems, while most credentialed psychologists from the same population train and practice in a Western, reductive medical model, which is often lacking in terms of real capacity for deep connection.

Now a successful and esteemed professional, Nile was walking through the market one day when a young man's face drew his attention. Nile could not stop himself from stopping dead in his tracks to stare. Not even when the young man lifted his head to lock eyes with him could Nile turn away because his heart had begun to swell in his chest. Slowly, recognition dawned on them both, and almost in slow motion, they started moving across the street toward each other.

"Nile?"

"Simon?"

It had been over 15 years since these brothers laid eyes on each other, Simon being a mere toddler when Nile was sent to sleep under his parents' house and then ran away. But as Caribbean people say, their blood pulled them toward each other. Brothers embraced in the center of the square, and both wept for joy.

"Look how beautifully you've grown!" Nile held his baby brother's face in his hands. "I have missed you more than words could ever say."

A blow caught Nile so hard on the side of his face that his cheek split and blood rushed out like Kaieteur falls. He lay on the pavement, dazed and confused, struggling to lift his head and clear his eyes. He heard his brother begin to scream and barely made out the words "No, Daddy! No!" before a savage boot caught him in the center of the same cheek and sent him rolling.

Nile's father thrust his face down close to his and spat at him, "Why didn't you just stay in the bush and die, faggot! I told you to stay away from us!" A crowd gathered and dragged the man off, as he dragged his youngest son behind him. Hands that Nile did not recognize picked him up and set him on his feet. "Lamb of God", he heard one woman say, genuine compassion in her voice "Lamb of God". Nile stumbled away, keeping his head down, shaken to the bone. Through sweat and blood-filled eyes, he found where he had parked his car and slid in. "You alright, son?" he heard passersby ask him. "You should go to the hospital. You took a bad one". But Nile drove himself as far from there as he could, to find himself at the edge of a waterfall's cliff where he had stood for many of his childhood years, trying to screw up the courage to dive headlong. He took his shoes off and stashed them neatly, prepared to send himself to his maker. "This Lamb of God, yes me. Take me. If you ever cared for me at all, take me now".

Many years later, Nile recounted to me that even as he leaned himself into the heavy wind that whipped the rivers around that part of the country, the wind seemed to push him back. Even as he leaned down toward the thunder of the falls crashing against the rocks below, the wind billowed in his face, literally holding him up and pushing him backward.

Eventually, exhausted, he gave up and lay down by the edge of the cliff, surrendering to whatever his destiny held in store. "I couldn't even lift my hand to wipe the spray from my eyes", he said. "I gave up completely". This is where his landscaping friends found him days later, as they had looked high and low for him after hearing about the scene in the market. They took him home, washed him down, and because he refused to go to any hospital, they brought him a nurse from a community clinic to sew up the nasty gash on his face.

In the days that passed, these friends treated Nile with the only painkillers they had, which resulted in Nile experiencing a very bad psychedelic trip. A drug-induced psychotic break ensued and friends now had no choice but to institutionalize him. Within this institution, the first-generation anti-psychotic medications that Nile was given caused his tongue to swell and his feet to shuffle, rendering him a complete mess of a man. It was Simon who came to his rescue, never having given up on reconnecting with his brother again, after that meeting in the market square. Simon signed him out of the facility into his own care, but then took Nile across the border to another place where he entered authentic rehabilitation. Simon's comforting reassurance was the first real soul-deep healing that Nile had felt since he was six years old, and he was now nearly 30.

I met Nile when he was in his mid-30s, when I was doing consultancy work for various UN agencies across the Caribbean and Latin America. Coincidentally, Nile's landscaping business had evolved to regional work as well. He was now commissioned for large-scale design, where he would envision multi-acre projects for resorts and large private estates, sketch them out, and train gardening staff before moving on to the next project. He would return several times over a two-year period to supervise and refresh the gardens in his care. Nile was in high demand and very well paid, but he only took on the projects he needed to sustain a quiet lifestyle and, more recently, to fund Simon's university education overseas.

Nile made the decision to marry a Ugandan woman to whom he had proposed within a few days of meeting. "It was like looking in a mirror", he said. "She has this shiny black skin like I have, and a massive scar running from left ear to right cheek. She wears a big, wide-brimmed straw hat and dark glasses, like I do, and doesn't like talking either. There's nothing really for us to say. We are grateful for life".

I was contracted by them to provide relationship counseling because Nile and his wife married each other for the specific purpose of protecting each other from even a sliver of future harm. "Not even an ant's bite", Neil said, yet they had the equal capacity to terrify each other half to death when flashbacks and nightmares came upon them, sometimes erupting in dangerous violence toward each other. We met, and continue to meet, either in person or by any number of the online platforms that came into practice during the COVID-19 lockdown. To stand and watch them walk away from a session, hand in hand, two large straw brims lifting gently in the breeze, is to fully take in the blissed privilege of working in this psychodynamic therapeutic vein.

In a recent research study conducted in the OECS – Organization of Eastern Caribbean States, the LGBTQI+ community is described as experiencing aggravated levels of ostracism, stigma, and discrimination because of their sexual orientation, and this translates into mental health disorders. Social isolation coupled with emotional and physical violence results in high rates of episodic and chronic mental illness, long-term depression, anxiety, and post-traumatic stress. Among MSM, drug and alcohol abuse are common as coping strategies, and they increase the likelihood of risky sexual behaviors. Lesbian and Bisexual Women face discrimination peculiar to them, including acts of gendered violence. They are also highly prone to drug use as a coping mechanism and to exacerbated mental health issues.

Negative mental health outcomes are worsened by the lack of mental health support for this demographic, homophobia from health service providers, and vulnerability to prosecution for private consensual behaviors. These laws and criminalizing behaviors "help create a context in which hostility and violence directed against LGBTQI+ people is legitimized, operating as an effective tool to ostracize and single out a vulnerable sector of the population" (Human Rights Watch).

In one island where large, numbers of MSM are victims of sexual violence and there is not enough real help for them, they will not report discrimination because of the criminalization of homosexuality, thus the silencing of many human rights violations experienced within the LGBTQI+ community.

LGBTQI+ people routinely face rape and sexual violence, criminalization, extortion, police violence and harassment, bullying, hate speech, denial of services and hampered access to justice. These violations, in and of themselves, are causal factors for poor mental health and well-being in the population, including anxiety, depression, traumatic stress, social isolation, and suicidality. However, when these "normal" mental health manifestations are left untended, they may amplify, embed, and evolve into more serious psychiatric concerns down the line. These may include Borderline states, Traumatic Stress Disorders, and Psychoses. Needless to say, these conditions may force school drop-outs, frequent sick leaves from jobs, and the active decline of a healthy, productive labor force. The quantifiable toll on economic systems is significant. State budgets normally allocated to mental health concerns are generally around 4% of the overall healthcare budget, which is up to 6% in some islands. In other words, mental health may receive 4% of 6% of a nation's annual budget. By comparison (though the comparison is with first world nations), note that Canada has a mental health care budget of $50 billion per year (Mental Health Commission Canada – MHCC), and the United Kingdom spends up to £64 billion annually.

It is also clear that women and girls in the Caribbean are affected by our region's rate of sexual activity involving minors under 13 years of age. As Now Grenada recently published, "sex crimes data indicates that men over the age of 50 are attracted to minors under 8" (April 2021). We have the second highest world rate of adolescent pregnancies which is a major contributor to poverty and to drop-out from formal education. In some Caribbean countries, the leading cause of maternal deaths is medical complications arising from unsafe abortions, particularly among adolescents, and this bears direct mental health consequences. The Caribbean also has the earliest age of sexual debut in the world, which often involves force. A significant portion of the victims (mostly girls) experience depression and suicidal ideation, along with more severe psychiatric disorders having their etiology in adverse childhood experiences.

For adult women, Intimate Partner Violence is the most significant and common danger. In Montserrat, for example, it is the most reported crime. Including sexual harassment, sexual violence, and sex/gender-based inequalities like unequal access to employment and sexual and reproductive health services, there is a pervasive and unrelenting mental health burden to carry.

Nevertheless, stigma and discrimination against mental health issues, stemming from inadequate understanding of what "mental health" is, mitigate against people in need seeking assistance. In the OECS, as in a significant proportion of the world population, there is a lack of understanding of the biological etiology of mental illness, and therefore, many groups attribute mental illness to supernatural forces and the enemy (Armiya'u & Adole, 2015). Most importantly, stigma and discrimination against key populations themselves, supported by legislation that is itself discriminatory, acts as an active barrier against members of vulnerable populations with mental health issues presenting for psychological or psychiatric care. In this culture, mental health workers reveal the lengths that individuals with emotional problems will go to, to *not* be discovered and treated, regardless of the depths of their suffering.

This is in keeping with international findings as well. According to the WHO, social stigma continues to be a barrier to seeking and receiving treatment for mental health difficulties. Carrying a label of mental illness does not only affect the person with the illness, but it can also affect family members and close friends, which in turn, can lead to a similar burden (known as courtesy stigma).

Because hate crimes and violence in targeted populations are under-reported throughout the OECS, provisions to assist this particular group are unidentified and lacking. There is therefore an inherent lack of psychosocial support, school counseling, and rehabilitation services for them. As such, there are a lot of people walking around being called "mad", and our culture is not providing any means of support. Legislation and policies need to speak to the protection of these people and once it does, legislation could even be considered preventive of mental health issues.

Manifestations of poor mental health in our marginalized populations often originate from discrimination within the legislative framework itself, rather than from organic medical conditions. Additionally, the very practice of Western psychiatry (including most psychologies and psychotherapies), which has been adopted as the preeminent "scientific" model, globally for over 300 years, has developed along racialized terms of reference, which themselves prove detrimental to constituents with different sexual orientations and gender identities, and who are vulnerable to various forms of silenced violence within the practice of mental health itself.

This is a deeply entrenched historical problem for the Caribbean. Added to concepts of mental health and well-being are the scars of imperial domination and persecution, during the era in which genocide, slavery, and colonialism flourished, as well as the effects of current economic oppression and indirect political control. "I am talking of millions of men who have been skillfully injected with fear, inferiority complexes, trepidation, servility, despair, and abasement" (Césaire, 1950).

In summary, multiple forms of human rights violations are perpetrated by discriminatory laws themselves, which affect expressions of sexual orientation and gender identity, cause poor mental health, and are impediments to overall well-being. Despite some good advances in some countries of the OECS, in others, there is no work on human rights, no refresher training for mental health professionals, no mental health information system, and no research or published articles on mental health.

Pulling from Paulo Freire's concept of *conscientization*, we integrate attitudes and perceptions from whole communities into social learning and social responsibilities regarding mental health and well-being rather than simply surveying and speaking to the handfuls of professionals currently working in our beleaguered region. Jung spoke of his own capacity for self-deceit when he consciously did not want to recognize something uncomfortable in a social setting, but the "eyes of the background", as he called it, always perceive when participation mystique blinds us to something about the group mind when it is not working in our individual best interest.

The Historical Development of Psychological Practice in the Caribbean and Latin America

The Caribbean is made up of 7,000 individual islands belonging to 28 separate island nations. In our 600-year-old history, counting from the time of European occupation, we have been colonized by England, France, Spain, Portugal, and Holland. Now, counting our Indigenous peoples, along with Africans, Indians, Asians, and other European groups such as Germans and Jews, we comprise over 50 sub-categories of ethnicities. Multicultural heritage is enshrined in our very existence. It is our cultural norm; the force that unites us. The islands share a common history of patriarchy, of strong adherence to religion with Catholicism being predominant, and a tradition of machismo, heterosexism, and extreme homophobia.

The case of Nile has illustrated some of the issues faced by key populations in their quest for psychological services and some of the dynamics encountered within the scope of a therapeutic relationship. Though diverse by nature, the Caribbean is a largely homophobic, patriarchal, hyper-masculine, heterosexist region. Here, instead of specialized psychological services that focus upon the depth and breadth of the needs of this population (inclusive of all those who come here to live, work, study, or play), like a trail through a forest that becomes fainter and fainter and finally seems to diminish to a nothing, traditional psychological theory too soon runs out for the creative, the gifted, the wounded and the deep.

General Psychological Services

Psychology and psychotherapy are relatively new fields to the region. They began to develop with the return home of nationals who had trained abroad, usually in the United Kingdom at that time. The University College of the West Indies in Jamaica was originally founded as an offshoot of the University of London in 1948. In the mid-1990s, psychology first appeared as an undergraduate program. Today, there are numerous university campuses and psychology training programs across the Caribbean, and in 2013, the Caribbean Alliance of National Psychological Associations – CANPA – was formed.

The favored psychological approach is overwhelmingly Cognitive Behavioral, as new colleges strive for accreditation and acclaim by sticking with the practices that appear most scientific. As the region grapples with such intense psychosocial issues as those discussed, along with among the highest rates of Child Sexual Abuse in the world (after sub-Saharan Africa and its tradition of child brides) and a startling frequency of national disasters such as hurricanes, earthquakes and floods, international donor agencies only support psychologies that are evidence-based, quantitative, relatively easy to administer and evaluate, and therefore usually of a CBT bent. However, "while we do have a good diagnostic statistical manual and a goodly amount of differential diagnosis, as well as the…parameters that define psychopathology through the organization in the psyche and the ego-self axis, there are yet other defining behaviors and feelings which…powerfully describe what is the matter" (Pinkola Estes, 1997, p. 11).

Psychoanalysis and the Depth Psychologies

In Argentina, by the 1980s, the psychoanalytic community was the fourth largest in the world, led only by America, France, and Germany. In Buenos Aires, home to 26 million people, there are more psychoanalysts than anywhere else in the world. In her journal article, Nancy Hollander described Argentina as an outpost for Spain during the colonial period. It soon became a haven for Italian, Irish, English, and other European settlers and was known as Latin America's most sophisticated, cosmopolitan, and wealthy capital.

The Argentine tango is one well-known art form aptly describing the ethos of the place, where 45% of the population was foreign-born. The dance, like the country, pivots on an axis of mourning for the homeland, the pain of an uprooted life, and betrayal in love. This population flocked to psychoanalysis, which knows well how to work with melancholia, loss, and mourning and which represented continental Europe's psychological foundations, thus being both mother and fatherland. Psychoanalysts became the most esteemed and privileged social class in Argentina, and when I attended a United Nations conference there, I was astonished by how many psychoanalysts' clinics existed within one city block, virtually side by side.

In the rest of Latin America, the tradition followed an established pattern for embedding psychoanalysis in the culture. There needs to be a highly professional training institute, regular conferences, and an exchange of international scholarship. Additionally, there needs to be publication of scientific papers, research, teaching, supervision, and ongoing advocacy for the new paradigm within the new culture. There also should be students who can afford the training, counting the luxuries of time and money, and clients who can pay to attend sessions several times a week for a period of years. In short, a stable, wealthy, intellectual, and Eurocentric society was required for the psychoanalytic tradition to take hold.

In Cuba, it was essentially the same, where the population was mainly comprised of Spaniards and Africans taken from their motherlands, albeit for opposite reasons. Exile is a common theme in Cuban art and literature, and other themes similar to those in Argentina emerged, including a clash of cultures, a rupture of social connections, and a dark chasm of loss and unfulfilled yearning. Following Castro's revolution in 1959, when many Cubans abandoned homes, property, businesses, and families to immigrate to America, the culture once again experienced a deep spiritual rupture, becoming a "site of incessant ideological conflict and … profound obscurity of meaning" (Edwin, 2004). Melancholia and mourning seeped into the culture's bones, and members of the Psychoanalytic Association of Cuba were kept running, managing both psychological and physical traumas of various kinds, including the wounds of war.

In Martinique, psychoanalysis established itself around an intellectual concept called *Antillanité*, a theory striving to assert itself against the doctrine of Negritude with its stress on African rather than Caribbean identity. Franz Fanon, a Martiniquan-born psychiatrist, is perhaps the most popular proponent of psychoanalysis in the French Caribbean, and other intellectuals, such as Eduard Glissant, joined him to establish a very short-lived psychoanalytic journal, 1971–1973. But here again, we see a similar trajectory of psychoanalytic roots forming around theoretical ideas in a demographic with wealth and stability enough to build the required blocks around a sustainable academic psychological movement.

In the Black, English-speaking Caribbean, however, psychoanalysis has not ventured.

Psychiatry in the Caribbean

The history of psychiatry and mental health in the Caribbean follows a similar path as the psychological. In the pre-colonial days, following the Indigenous, community-based model, people with mental health disorders were treated "with salient herbs which were blended with food … and by the administration of unguents and lavings while singing. They were treated without restraints and with rudimentary attempts at pharmacology and cultural therapies" (Hickling, n.d.).

During the period of slavery, while doctors looked after the local white population, medical attention for all patients, particularly the slaves, was impossible. Black slave preachers and obeah men filled the gap, being almost entirely independent of white control. They contributed enormously to the physical and psychological well-being of the slaves and had so much influence throughout society that British authorities introduced draconian legislation banning the use of obeah across the Caribbean (Hickling, n.d.).

Then, in accordance with the British model, psychiatric institutions – more often referred to as "lunatic asylums" and "mad houses," – were established in many islands between 1850 and 1900. These asylums were places where the mentally ill could be kept under custodial institutionalization or locked away from society for many years or even forever.

With the gradual introduction of psychotherapeutic treatments and the arrival of psychiatric pharmacotherapy, several countries and territories started developing services for the mentally ill in the community as they sought alternative ways to treat people outside of large asylums. Many countries and territories are engaged in the process of deinstitutionalization and the development of community-based mental health services.

Currently, this initiative has slowed down, and it is mainly the centralized services that remain. (There are anomalies, such as in Antigua, where services have almost all been decentralized and returned to a community base). Today, significant work has been achieved in terms of understanding state responsibility toward mental health services in the Caribbean. Note, however, that several states have not acknowledged the difference between policies and plans, the practice result being that while much research and academic work has been done, a system of praxis has not followed, and little real change has, in fact, occurred.

Today, in 2023, it is fair to say that both the training of psychologists and the practice of psychology are coming more and more in alignment with the needs of society as it has evolved; the road has been long, and the standard, Western, medical model in practice is still the one preferred, by far.

References

Armiya'u AY, & Adole O. (2015). Relationship between sociodemographic characteristics, psychiatric burden and violent offence in a maximum security prison in North-Central Nigeria. *Journal of Forensic Science & Criminology 3*(2), 202. https://doi.org/10.15744/2348-9804.2.502

Avert. (2019). *HIV and AIDS in Latin America, the Caribbean Regional Overview.* https://www.avert.org/professioinals/hiv-around-world/latin-america/overview

Bagley, C., & D'Augelli, A. R. (2000). Suicidal behavior in gay, lesbian, and bisexual youth: It's an international problem that is associated with homophobic legislation. *British Medical Journal, 320*, 1617–1618. https://doi.org/10.1136/bmj.320.7250.1617

Brewster, F. (2020). *The Racial Complex: A Jungian Perspective in Culture and Race.* Routledge.

Brooks, J. (2015). *Learning from the Lifeworld.* The British Psychological Society. https://www.bps.org.uk/psychologist/learning-lifeworld

Césaire, A. (1950). Discourse on Colonialism. Les Classiques. No. 391.

De Graff, R., Sandfort, T., & Have, M. (2006). Suicidality and sexual orientation: Differences between men and women in a general population-based sample from the Netherlands. *Archives of Sexual Behavior, 35*, 253–262. https://doi.org/10.1007/s10508-006-9020-z

Edwin, S. (2004). *Cultural Healing: Gender, Race, and Trauma in Literature of the Americas.* PhD thesis. Stony Brook University, New York

Frankl, V. (2000). *Man's Search for Ultimate Meaning.* Perseus Publishing.

Morrison, T. (2017). *The Origin of Others.* Harvard University Press.

Von Franz, M. (1990). *Alchemy.* Inner City Books.

Chapter 7

Maddinks the Mute

Fana watched the seaweed ebb and flow. It was bright orange in color, dendrites floating off in every direction like a big skirt, billowing and folding in, inviting and receding. Fana wished she could float off like that. To become Sargassum weed and exist way out in the ocean, unbothered, untouched, eventually to sink to the bottom in peaceful repose. But for today, it was the dusty streets again. Rickety cars, open convertibles, and dark-windowed sedans blasting reggae, rap, and gospel at competing intensity. The roads were littered with plastic Coke bottles, discarded Kentucky Fried Chicken (KFC) boxes, sweetie wrappers, and cigarette butts. Dogs snapped and snarled at each other, fighting for bones and scraps in adjacent alleyways.

Fana's mother looked down and adjusted the talisman hanging from a leather thong around her daughter's neck. Her eyes were bloodshot from sleeplessness, and her feet were blistered and bare, but she had taken her child and left. This time, she would keep going.

"Maddinks!" someone called at her from across the road. "Maddinks! Where you think you going again? They coming for you g'yal, they coming!" Maddinks put a hustle in her step. She had run away from the House of the Rising Sun several times before, wrapping her waist-long locks up into a tall head tie. Each time she ran away, the pastor sent a van to pick her up and take her back via the Mental.

"Screeeeee!" Maddinks called back at the man. "Screeeeeee!" She had given up language at an early age, responding with eerie stillness and blank stares to initiations of conversations from others. A visiting professional from the Peace Corps suggested mutism, a form of schizophrenia, and the suggestion stuck with the community, who promptly supplied the more explicitly local term, "Dummy". Going from Dummy to the more elevated "Maddinks" in her adolescence, she never moved to refute it. She simply left people to believe what they wanted and let the assumptions fly. She understood clearly that the labels and stigmatizations associated with her apparent disability, perceived mental instability, and the social bullying that went with them were more representative of the "eye of the beholder" than her own truth.

Maddinks had grown up in a residential home for the disabled but was treated so horribly there that at age 16, she left to volunteer for a different brand of trouble

DOI: 10.4324/9781003223603-9

in the House of the Rising Sun, a religious community high up in the hills. The compound overlooked a picturesque cityscape teaming with bustle, dust, and noise. The vast Atlantic rolled in the distance, and behind the compound, the forest rose. Within a year, Maddinks had borne a child by the head pastor; an initiation of sorts, she was led to believe. But now, as their daughter, Fana, blossomed into puberty and the pastor started giving his own offspring "that look", Maddinks began to make her moves. Three failed run-away attempts, each costing her a lengthy, punitive stay in The Mental, prompted her to learn to strategize more carefully.

Maddinks had her first nervous breakdown within the mental health institution, a direct result of the force they applied when she refused to adhere to their medication regimen. Subsequent involuntary hospitalizations could then easily be orchestrated by the pastor, in which he would report "unstable and dangerous behavior", and police would arrive to handcuff Maddinks and drag her off. Deemed incompetent to make her own decisions and prone to running off with "that poor child" in tow, Maddinks lived under perpetual threat of being institutionalized and heavily drugged again if she were non-compliant with the expectations of the pastor and his flock. Worse, she was consistently threatened with having her child taken away from her for the very reason of her attempts to flee the compound and, as they charged, "exposing the child to the dangers of homelessness". So, at the institution, where they mistook her refusal to speak for an intellectual disability, she let them think so while she made her plans on the literal quiet.

This is the second of two black, female, impoverished, and disabled victims of child sexual abuse that I describe in this text, both of whom suffered acute mental health breakdown. It provides an opportunity to speak of the female voice, or feminist voice, and all of the varied ways in which women may vocalize to make themselves heard and understood. This is urgent to address from cultural and political points of view, but within the context of this narrative, I will mainly focus upon the psychological. But even as I write this, is it not clear that the psychological is itself the cultural and the political? As Fanon asserts, any presumed dichotomy between the psychological and the political is false.

In the case of Elusine, she told us that her daughter, though she did not form recognizable words, instead made sounds that were recognizably expressive of specific emotions. In psychotherapy, a professional leans into the therapeutic encounter, "listening in" for the gestures, postures, utterances, and other indicators that provide meaning. Jungian Psychology brings word association, dream analysis, projective tests, sand play therapy, and other approaches that allow the workings of the unconscious to come to light. Psychology, being a discipline of interiority, clients are often taken aback to find that sessions are far from an exercise in intellectual jousting, but instead are a sincere foray into the workings of the unconscious via numerous means as well as speech. In her essay "The Transformation of Silence into Language and Action", Audre Lorde (2007) writes:

> I am standing here as a Black Lesbian poet … I am still alive, and might not
> have been … I have come to believe over and over again that what is most

important to me must be spoken, made verbal and shared, even at the risk of having it bruised or misunderstood ... What are the words you do not yet have? What do you need to say? What are the tyrannies you swallow day by day and attempt to make your own until you sicken and die, still in silence?

(Lorde, 2007, pp. 40–41)

And again, in a dialogue with her daughter about the transformation of silence, Lorde's daughter said:

Tell them about how you're never really a whole person if you remain silent, because there's always that one little piece inside you that wants to be spoken out, and if you keep ignoring it, it gets madder and madder, and if you don't speak it out one day it will just jump up and punch you in the mouth from the inside.

(Lorde, 2007, p. 43)

In this gathering of stories, when Melanie, Yusuf, Yara, Elusine, Maddinks, and Bahira trusted enough or were desperate enough to speak, their sound was labeled either psychotic or devil-possessed, and they shut down again, more traumatized than before. In the case of Maddinks, she eventually cultivated a unique language of her own alongside a close community of artists who joined her in making the music of the trance. Together, they marshaled a spectrum of collective voices speaking nothing of aggression, darkness, or disease but instead urging listeners to health, freedom, and the power lying untapped within their own souls.

While resident on the compound of the Rising Sun, Maddinks began to orchestrate the ritual release of physical and spiritual restraint for the women in her circle; those that she recognized to feel as trapped and hopeless as herself. Maddinks unconsciously drew from the African and Indigenous spiritualist traditions that existed in her multi-ethnic lineage to curate ceremonial dance as a means of throwing off the shackles of oppression and fear and taking up more organic self-empowerment in the process. She became a master conductor in her own silent manner, knew how to mediate the energies of those coming under her direction, and her reputation as a healer grew.

Maddinks choreographed her ceremonies with her heart set on revolution, though she may not herself have chosen that word. Whether the gatherings were called Santeria, voodoo, candomblé, or church, her intention was to unravel the totalitarian state in which the pastor kept the residents subservient to his will, being aware that he was merely a symbol of patriarchal, colonialist, and male-dominated power systems. He acted as he had been programmed, never an original idea in his head, and personified the absolute confidence of a man who had never even contemplated losing power.

Fanon wrote that any study of the colonial world needs to take into consideration the phenomena of ecstatic dance and possession. He wrote, "The purpose in coming together is to allow the ... hampered aggressivity to dissolve as in a volcanic eruption ... one step further and you are completely obsessed" (Fanon, p. 45). Note that this has direct application to Dionysus and Jab-Jab as well, as we will see in the case of Vladimir. But in this case, Maddinks proved herself the direct opposite of the pastor, who spoke from the front of many shelves of pretty books and wielded his words like daggers, slicing away at the confidence of his congregation, carving shame, indebtedness, and dependency out of their cores. He had an over-big suit, an over-big head, and was fully corrosive in his practice.

On the other hand, Maddinks carried the archetypes of anarchist, architect, and politician, and she did all of her work without the benefit of speech. Instead, she embodied compassion, wisdom and healing grace, and she nurtured power in her blood, her soul, and her drum.

When Jung searched for the psychogenesis of spiritualistic phenomena within the scope of the mind, he discovered that African and Indigenous peoples understood spirit possession to be firmly rooted in the corps; in the physical body. In Maddinks, body and mind coalesced. Similarly to Jung, Lorde would also have described this as a "non-European consciousness of living" (2007, p. 37) in which, for women, neither dance, music nor connection with the spirit world are luxuries nor is it suspicious, but is a vital necessity of existence. Lorde wrote, "It forms the quality of the light within which we predicate our hopes and dreams toward survival and change, first made into language then into ideas then into more tangible action" (2007, p. 37). Lorde tells us that for each of us as women, within our deep, dark spaces, we hold phenomenal creativity and power.

In Maddinks' new world, the pastor, ever-present bible in hand, peeped upon these ceremonies that Maddinks led and could not fail to acknowledge her charismatic hold over those seeking her interventions. He told her, "I empower you to conduct the ceremonies". Maddinks marveled at the absurdity of his belief that all the power she contained had been bestowed by him. But she dropped her eyes in acquiescence and went her silent way; this man was not one to aggravate, his wickedness defied imagination. She dropped her eyes, smiled her "crazy" smile, and strategized.

Maddinks believed wholeheartedly in the one God, but the spirits abiding in the realm of the ancestors always felt more accessible to her. She felt a deep connection with them, as though they came immediately whenever she called, so Maddinks kept around her all of the things her spirits would like to make them feel welcomed and at home. The dichotomy between Maddinks and the pastor represents many dualities: sacred vs profane, masculine vs feminine, and formal psychological processes vs indigenous practice. Ultimately, however, Maddinks worked to dissolve the polarities and render herself and her clientele unified as one.

Memory and the Body

Maddinks' system operated on several different psychosomatic levels, taking memory and the body as just one example. In 2022, Gentsch published an article titled *Clinical Manifestations of Body Memories: The Impact of Past Bodily Experience on Mental Health*. Taking from cognitive neuroscience and clinical neuroscience, they wrote that bodily experiences activate brain networks that mediate higher-order processing. Negative body memories contribute to the development of mental health problems. Past violence, anger, and fear, while not always accessible to conscious reflection, may impact our bodily states at any given time. Sigmund Freud, Sandor Ferenczi, and Merleau-Ponty have also written about this, drawing mainly from the field of neurology. Their literature is too vast to synthesize in the context of this narrative, but in the context of victims of trauma, such as the cases presented here, Gentsch wrote that "trauma memory is used by clinical psychologists and psychiatrists to describe the encoding of past traumatic life events involving fear of death and other serious bodily threats" (Gentsch, 2022, 2.1). To put it in layman's terms, Maddinks aimed to shake the encoded memories of these threats and fears loose and reencode new narratives along new neural pathways that spoke only of kindness, freedom, and power.

Traumatic body memories are mainly observed in patients with Post Traumatic Stress Disorder (PTSD), including memories of pain under torture, pain under sexual assault, or pain from an acute injury such as a vehicular accident. For child trauma victims, the re-enactment of a frightening event has been observed as a frequent consequence even years later, as we have discussed in the context of Jung's ideas on repetition compulsion in the cases of Yusuf and Vladimir.

Indigenous cultures have long developed rituals for coping with traumatic release from the body. In this tradition, the body is the central actor in both sensing and managing emotions. Dance serves to invite patterns of engagement with other bodies as they move within relational space in which emotions are explored, articulated, and reworked.

Without a day of formal study in trauma releasement techniques, Maddinks accessed the collective wisdom and experiences of her ancestral practices and discovered herself an intuitive master of the organic healing arts.

Some distance from the compound where she and Fana lived was an extensive forest. Like her own mother before her, Maddinks often took her daughter on long walks through it, foraging for medicinal plants and fruits from trees that had sprung up randomly, where a wayfarer spat out seeds that almost instantly rooted. On these excursions, Maddinks felt in close proximity to the natural energies that sustained her, and it was only here that she allowed herself to vocalize. At the foot of one tree, she'd leave an offering for the spirit of that tree; some wildflower she'd gathered along the way. Often, she stood still and sang a song to the spirit, and as Fana took in the emotion behind the song that she sang, she realized her mother was offering a comfort to the spirits; that she did not feel subservient to them but on par. As Maddinks honored the power of the spirit world, so did that world open up to show her the divinity within herself. Whenever other villagers were on the outskirts of the forest as Maddinks emerged, they saw her face to be luminous, her posture erect, her stride determined and forthright. "Crazy woman", they whispered. "Mad as a hatter". And from a safe, silly distance they chanted, giggling, "Maddinks, Maddinks, Maddinks!"

Fana would feel her mother tighten the grip on her hand and they'd walk faster. Anger swelled in Maddinks, enraged that no one cared that they were obliging an innocent child to witness her mother bullied and humiliated in public. Fana felt the anger and the shame as though it poured into her via an umbilical storm. In fact, Fana had experienced these feelings of shame and embarrassment from birth, or if possible, from before. No celebrations accompanied her delivery, just a quick mop-up of her mother, a quick wipe-down of herself, and a rough admonition to "do better!" No presents accompanied any of her birthdays nor did medals accompany her wins at sports. There was never a comfort but her mother's perpetual finger under her chin, lifting her head and indicating with a worried smile, "Keep your head up, child. Head up".

What Maddinks could not convey to her child is that she was purposefully using her time "under" the pastor to their ultimate benefit. She understood that if she allowed herself to become subservient to the authority of the elders, who certainly recognized her inherent power, they would find a way to capture and subvert her gift. As Fanon expressed concerning the manner in which settler colonialism affects its subjects, one is not merely displaced from one's land but from one's rightful mind.

Settler colonialism is a patriarchal and gendered process in which settlers seek to displace, drive away, and eliminate or "violently depopulate" indigenous peoples. "Ordinary" colonialism, on the other hand, simply aims to control and economically exploit those existing on the land without the colonists themselves necessarily wanting to live there. This phenomenon has been in the world since Europe established colonies in Africa, Asia, and the Americas in the 16–20th centuries. As Asante pointed out (2016), similar to both Fanon and Buber, the seizing and displacement of peoples from land also involves the colonization and displacement of minds.

While those in Maddinks the Mute's religious community sought to make a name for themselves by preying on the worst fears of superstitious congregants, claiming to chase out ghosts and other malevolent entities, they had to admit that their reputation and success in the community was lukewarm at best, and their coffers were dwindling. They recognized that Maddinks appealed to the highest rather than lowest denominators. People came to her for herbal remedies, bone broths, music and dance, and the liberatory movements of her releasement ceremonies. Her personal power seemed to be on the rise, her healing skills now including production values like setup and organization along with integrity, humility and talent. When she led ceremony, people came in droves from all around, walking through the jungle at night in ones, twos, and larger groups, seeing only by the light of their cellular phones. And, as she provided no words; no sermon, so to speak, no charges could be imposed upon the intentions of Maddinks the Mute.

Maddinks had been raped several times, all under the age of ten, before she was removed from her family of origin and institutionalized as an abused, neglected, and abandoned child. She would now rather die than give people any more of herself than she allowed. Each time she recalled the words of the man who had laid down on her body and whispered into her brain, "Tell me you like it. You like it, don't you? Say it!", she vowed to never let her speech become occupied. She vowed that no mortal would hear a single word from her tongue, including the child she later bore by the same violent means. She was a new type of scholar now, with a new type of ontology, a hauntologist, as Rahimi might say. People felt healed and freed by her, simply via the force of her presence, her baraka.

One day, a new man came. He said he was an anthropologist from a university in America, and he wanted to write about Fana's mother. Fana intervened on Maddink's behalf. "She doesn't speak", she told the man. "At least not to other people". The man turned toward Maddinks in an unhurried, soft-gazing way. "Tell me your name" he said. A jolt went through Fana's body, but it passed through like surf billowing across the shore. Her entire being understood that something had instantly changed. Following the man's gaze, she turned to her mother and saw her as if for the first time.

Her mother was an even mix of African and Middle Eastern. She always kept her head covered but underneath the scarf her hair was fat. It curled here, kinked there, and flattened out straight in cool weather. When she loosened her braids for brushing, they expanded like great oceans reaching back for ancestral shores. Mother's lips were fat too, Fana thought, as were her breasts. And her eyes, regarding the man through half-lowered lids, now processed an alchemical transformation. My mother is phenomenally beautiful, Fana thought. Rather, she is a phenomenon. And to put a star on the tree of this new situation, Mother opened her mouth and answered the man. "I am Fana".

How bizarre, her daughter thought, to have given me her own name. What does it mean? Things moved quickly from there.

The man, whose name was Fassil and who was quiet, kind, and thoughtful, acquired some land and built a small cabin in just over six months. There was room for the three of them, and the rooms were safe and airy. Mother Fana spent her time much as she always had, foraging for wild plants and flowers in the days and conducting ceremony most nights. Participants now came from overseas as well as from the region; the pastor and his community left far behind. Fassil walked beside Mother Fana. Everywhere she went, he went too, carrying her bags, photographing her flowers, stroking her hair. In between, he wrote and wrote on his pages. He wrote and cooked food. Ox-tail stew, fresh hot bread with butter and fried onions, heaps of green salads and green beans, and Middle Eastern spices from the Syrian and Lebanese souks. It was good.

"But I don't want to be like you, Mama" Fana said one day. Mother Fana and her new husband took this in quietly, as was their manner. And as was Fassil's way, he made arrangements with calm efficiency. Within the year, Fana the child was packed to leave for America, where she would spend some time with Fassil's parents in upstate New York in preparation for university qualifications.

The path from Fassil and Mother Fana's house was unpaved and uneven. It took a few minutes to walk from the front porch to the taxi, and as she walked, Fana heard her mother start to sing. She stopped a while to listen, her head turned to the sound, and she felt it cascade upon her skin as rain. Mother was singing protection upon her, one hand waving goodbye, the other on her rising belly where a new life was turning.

Fana did not look back. She could see very clearly with other than eyes; speak very clearly with other than words. I am your descendent, Mama, she conveyed. I am the whole bloodline. Your heart beats in my chest. Shukran.

The taxi driver put his hand on the horn and gestured at his watch. Fana got in and sped away to new beginnings.

The Cultural Dimensions of Spirit Possession

Mankind has always been fascinated by the metaphysical and supernatural. Whether we adore or fear it or indifferently acknowledge that it is there but benign, we are fascinated by the existence of a world that can neither be seen nor subjected to empirical evidence (Amin et al., 2006). In various parts of the Mediterranean, West and Central Asia, Northern Africa, and Latin and South America, there is a strong belief in the "Evil Eye". This refers to a vindictive look which is believed to be able to cause harm upon another person (Rassool, 2018). Many of these cultures craft amulets, lockets, talismans, and other protective objects to ward off the evil eye, which they hang in their homes and cars or wear on their bodies (Pew Research Centre, 2022). In Persia, Morocco, Iraq, Saudi Arabia, and many other Arab states, elaborate rituals involving the burning of various seeds and herbs are performed, and Turkish Airlines has a protective emblem painted on their planes. Similarly, in several parts of Africa protective symbols are worked into wall hangings and jewelry, and in India black Kohl is used around the eyes or on the forehead. Some religions have prayers that are especially invoked to rid oneself of possession by the unseen.

However, despite the significant size of this global community of individuals who seek psychological assistance for these matters of non-material interference, many psychologists who are trained in the Western empiricist approach regard complaints of spirit possession as a clinical enigma and prefer to turn their backs on this population for fear of not being taken seriously themselves. Clinging hard to scientism – the notion that the scientific worldview is the only one, they dismiss the client with "That is just superstitious nonsense". On the other side of the coin are psychologists and other mental health professionals who do share these beliefs but keep them hidden, for the same fear of offending scientism, yet they unskillfully project their fears upon clients who otherwise might find a sound psychological path to understanding.

And, along with cultural, collective ontologies defining how individual psychologists and other practitioners regard the notion of the spirit world, there is also the individual personality driving individual practitioners' stance. Take the trait of "Openness" in the Five Factor model, for example. Openness is defined as being creative, imaginative, curious, psychologically minded, and flexible in thinking. In contrast, individuals who score low in this dimension tend to shy away from the unfamiliar, and to refute experiences outside of their own worldviews.

Mental health professionals who score low on the openness scale, and who have not done the necessary reflective work on how their personal core beliefs may affect relationships with clients, are more likely to disparage belief systems that are unlike their own, consciously or unconsciously.

In 1997, Maya Angelou wrote of our society's fear of indigenous African beliefs, and not much has changed since then. She wrote, "There is one major explanation for the old negative image of Africa and all things African held by so many. Slavery's profiteers had to convince themselves and their clients that the persons they enslaved were little better than beasts ... (they) had to persuade slave buyers that the African was a primitive, a cannibal, and richly deserved oppression. How else could the Christian voice be silent – how soothe the Christian conscience?" (Angelou, 1997, pp. 14–16). The slaves soon began to believe what their masters believed: Africa was a continent of savages. Even in religious matters ... most failed to see the correlation between the African and his gris-gris (religious amulets) and the Muslim with this beads or the Catholic with his rosary. This internalization of victimhood works at societal level and on individual level as well, unless and until there is organized resistance. This is a phenomenon that we are seeing play out in Israel's genocide of the Palestinians today, as with the individual perpetrators of abuse carried out by the males and females in this text.

Possession in the African Caribbean: Religion, Superstition, and Calling Down the Spirits

Christianity is the largest religion in the world, at 31.5% of the population, followed by Islam at 23.2%, Hinduism at 15%, Buddhism at 7.1% and Judaism at 0.2%. These are the "big five". Additionally, Chinese traditional religions account for 394 million people in the world, Primal-Indigenous 300 million, and African/Diasporic 100 million. The Caribbean and Latin American region is known as one of the most religious territories in the world where its religions also include Rastafarianism, Voodoo, Santeria, Obeah, Shango, Orisha and more, along with the "big five". This gives rise to many complex contestations about religious practice and the "coloniality of power", including issues of ethnic identity and human rights (Campbell & Se-Wheatle, 2020). Generally speaking, disruptions to the established order of religion or the law are not condoned, with religion playing a key role in legal discussions and decisions around sex, sexuality, reproductive rights, and gender. In this arena, some African and Indian spiritual practices are legally forbidden (Paton, 2015; Rocklin, 2015; Boaz, 2017). "Colonial regulation of Obeah through laws dating as far back as 1760 continues to suppress African and immigrant religious practices, ensuring that the coloniality of power pervades Caribbean societies well into the twenty-first century" (Campbell & Wheatle, 2020). This translates into a clear pattern of racialized hierarchies in psychology as well as in religion and law. Culture and religion have significant influences on the diagnoses and prevalence of psychological disorders, particularly psychosis in children. In psychiatry, there has always been a dichotomy between religion and mental health, with "possession usually perceived and labeled as psychotic disorders" (Rassool, 2018, p. 24).

Counter-Hegemonic Discourse

A part of the Caribbean complexity includes the fact that these very populations, with their indigenous roots in deeply cultured places, do acknowledge, make space for, and hold the ancestral spirits dear. But possession by spirits other than Christian spirits is where they all balk, however, as fear of the demonic (read "anything non-Christian") is as old and as international as antiquity.

> A most curious phenomenon of the personality, one which has been observed for centuries but which has not yet received its full explanation, in that in which the individual seems to be the vehicle of a personality that is not his own. Someone else's personality seems to "possess" him and to be finding expression through his words and actions, whereas the individual's own personality is temporarily "lost" or "gone". This happens with all degrees of malignancy. There seem to be all degrees of the same basic process from the simple, benign observation that so-and-so "takes after her father", or "that's her mother's temper coming out in her", to the extreme distress of the person who finds himself under a compulsion to take on the characteristics of a personality he may hate and/or feel to be entirely alien to his own.
>
> (Laing & Esterson, 1990, p. 58)

It is fair and understandable, all things considered, to acknowledge that if you feel you risk being taken over by a demonic entity, you would be afraid to go there. But what of the field of psychology? What is its responsibility, especially considering the victims of violence described in this text? One way, evidently, is dissociation and avoidance within the profession itself. Western psychology that operates in a purely medical model has learned to keep religion and the spiritual out of psychological work. However, Jungian psychology knows that it is impossible.

Pastors inherently understand the entanglement between psychology and religion, and in terms of Child Abuse Psychosis, they recognize the symptoms. Where a psychiatrist would go toward anti-psychotic medications and treatments without addressing underlying psychological issues, pastors exorcise demons, without pursuing their realm of origin. Both are right and both are wrong.

In America, where African Americans reportedly have a greater severity of untreated mental health disorders than any other known racial group (Dempsey et al., 2016), this demographic has been found more likely to rely on the elders of their churches and their own spiritual beliefs than mental health professionals. This is because of the distrust that accompanies institutionalized racism in America and psychology's historic inattention to cultural issues in the application of diagnostics and treatment planning. Additionally, potential clients fear the profession's propensity to misdiagnose due to stereotypical and social media-based ideas of the population.

Churches and religion have become the spinal cord of diasporic African peoples the world over, including the Caribbean, where slavery and oppression needed a safe haven for seeking emotional refuge, expressing authentic feelings, performing important rituals, and building the foundations of community. Helping resources like after-school tutoring became the source of healing for psychological issues as well. While stigmas exist against mental illness and seeking psychological help, going to church remains encouraged and heroic. Plus, it is free, does not require health insurance, does not usually have long waiting lists, and singing prayer has always been cathartic for believers.

After Hurricane Katerina in New Orleans, Black pastors began to advise their parishioners to seek psychological services from outside agencies, as their significantly higher level of distress could not be met by the church (Dempsey et al., 2016). In Grenada, after Hurricanes Ivan and Emily (2005, 2006) the magnitude of the disaster and people's desperation for help led to a significant uptake of the psychological services provided by the United Nations. It marked the turning point in recognition of the helpfulness of the profession, despite some stigmas still remaining deeply entrenched. That is, the population would now seek psychological help, but usually keep it down-low.

These disasters have marked a turning point in how the field of psychology is incorporated into the warp and weft of daily life, how it is taught by educators, and how it is applied by new practitioners who come out of the same cultural soup as those afflicted and needing help. I believe that we are on the cusp now, of something truly relevant to these times.

References

Amin, A., Gadit, M., & Callanan, T. S. (2006) Jinni possession: A clinical enigma in mental health. *The Journal of the Pakistan Medical Association, 56*(10), 476–478. https://www.jpma.org.pk/PdfDownload/894

Angelou, M. (1997). *Even the Stars look Lonesome*. Random House.

Boaz, D. (2017). Obeah, vagrancy, and the boundaries of religious freedom: Analyzing the proscription of "pretending to possess supernatural powers" in the Anglophone Caribbean. *Journal of Law and Religion, 32*(3), 423–448. https://doi.org/10.1017/jlr.2017.44

Campbell, Y., & Se-Wheatle, S. (2020). Contradictions in faith in the Caribbean context: Postcolonialism, religion, and the constitution. *Commonwealth & Comparative Politics, 58*(3), 277–284. https://doi.org/10.1080/14662043.2020.1782624

Dempsey, K., Butler, S. K., & Gaither, L. (2016). Black churches and mental health professionals: Can this collaboration work? *Journal of Black Studies, 47*(1), 73–87. http://www.jstor.org/stable/24572960

Gentsch, A. (2022). Clinical manifestations of body memories: The impact of past bodily experiences on mental health. *Brain Sciences, 12*(5), 594. https://doi.org/10.3390/brainsci12050594

Laing, R. D., & Esterson, A. (1970). *Sanity, Madness, and the Family*. Pelican Books.

Lorde, A. (2007). *Sister Outsider*. Crossing Press.

Paton, D. (2015). *The Cultural Politics of Obeah: Religion, Colonialism and Modernity in the Caribbean World*. Cambridge University Press. https://doi.org/10.1017/CBO9781139198417

Pew Research Center. (2022, May 10). *Chapter 4: Other beliefs and practices*. Pew Research Center's Religion & Public Life Project. https://www.pewresearch.org/religion/2012/08/09/the-worlds-muslims-unity-and-diversity-4-other-beliefs-and-practices/

Rassool, G. H. (2018). *Evil Eye, Jinn Possession, and Mental Health Issues: An Islamic Perspective*. Routledge.

Rocklin, A. (2015). Obeah and the politics of religion's making and unmaking in colonial Trinidad. *Journal of the American Academy of Religion, 83*(3), 697–721. https://doi.org/10.1093/jaarel/lfv022

Chapter 8

Elusine

Elusine had remarkable intelligence in herbal medicines. She grew everything she needed on the hillside at the back of her home. Farming that steep incline had given her enviable physical strength as well, and as she rested between digging the soil and harvesting produce, she would look out upon the sea where Atlantic surf relentlessly pounded Caribbean shores and find cause for peacefulness and joy. When I visited her, it was as much to provide psychosocial services as it was to give myself a respite. Elusine always had something unusual to offer, like soup made from watermelons, tamarinds, or other fruits. "Not juice", she would affirm, "It's hot soup with peppers and herbs. Good for the constitution". If she put chicken in anything, it was feet and necks. If beef, it was tripe, tail, or tongue. Sometimes, it was simply green-fig and olive oil or green-fig and butter. Crix and cheese was a treat. Elusine loved to laugh and had a nuanced joie de vivre that I immensely enjoyed. Yet, never once had she passed a basic mental health status exam. Her sanity met her madness around the edges like the Atlantic met the Caribbean. Sometimes, the collision was a churning, chaotic mess of white emotional foam, but sometimes, crazy greeted sane like the deep kiss from an old lover, one you simultaneously kept at arm's length but felt bound to for all time.

When grounded in the immediate present, she could name all of her herbs, what they would cure, and under which moon they should best be harvested. She knew all the possible side effects of each and how to counteract any ill effects. She recommended dosages, whether leaves should best be consumed dried or in tea, and what each plant's stem, flower, or bark yielded. But sometimes, caught in the sudden shadow of some dark cloud falling, she would lose track, lose time, lose all sensible cognition, and begin to narrate stories that held no coherence except for a running thread of unbearable anguish.

Elusine had fled the island to seek betterment in Venezuela when she was a skinny adolescent girl with hair the color of bronze, following a promise of employment as a housekeeper there. She had fled the island because she'd been trapped as her father's sex slave from the age of five, her father being of particularly brutal temperament, her mother and siblings all incapable of intervention. But once in Venezuela, she continued to be raped by her employers until she found herself pregnant, and they threw her out with no working papers and a new daughter in

DOI: 10.4324/9781003223603-10

tow, black-skinned and blue-eyed. Thanks to Elusine's stubborn determination to make something safe of her life, she returned to the island of her birth with savings enough to purchase a small plot of rocky hillside and slowly built a very modest structure for herself and her child. She earned a sufficient living by selling her produce at the market and dedicated the remainder of her life to the ferocious protectiveness of her child.

The child had been born without the power of speech. Doctors said she had perfect hearing and no medical reason for an impediment, but nevertheless, she did not ever talk. She made sounds, and as her mother said, the sounds were not to be interpreted as signifiers for words but as expressions of emotion. Thus, the child expressed an abundance of joy, surprise, amazement, and compassion, the emotions with which she had been raised. Because of her blue eyes and black skin, villagers nicknamed her "Jet Blue", and because she did not use language, they decided she had bad spirits in her. Her mother only laughed out loud at them. "Yes", she said, "That's right. She's anointed. Stay far".

Elusine suffered from acute paranoia. Amulets to repel the evil eye swung from her ceiling on lengths of twine, and bowls of holy water sat on the floor in all corners. In her garden, she tied the ends of long grass together in the evenings, forming a kind of lasso that would catch your feet and send you flying if you came sneaking up at night. She strung the thinnest strands of fishing line between trees at neck length, invisible in the darkness, waiting to garrot any incoming enemies. Around and about her rickety house was one trap after the other for strangers, yet if Elusine welcomed you in, she treated you like gold.

She met a man one day, and after some time of courtship, she allowed him to visit her at home and then to stay over and move in. She told me he had such a permanently apologetic look on his face that she foresaw no danger. But a year or so into their domestic arrangement, Elusine was awoken at night by the sound of grief coming from her child. "She squabbled", Elusine told me. "Grief came out of her like a squabble of barking dogs. It seized my heart".

Through a series of sounds, gestures, and putting-it-together, it was discovered that the apologetic man had raped the girl child numerous times, always anally, to avoid either detection or pregnancy. The girl had only cried out when she finally could take it no more.

The police descended on the house in no time flat due to the almighty noise that Elusine made in the dead of night and due to neighbors' frantic reporting that she was chasing her boyfriend down the hill, machete swinging left and right.

A court case quickly ensued, as there was no doubt about what had transpired. In my role, I faced the unbearable reality that I could not help Elusine hold her mind together, fragile as it already was, in the face of the defense attorney's hammering. Worse, she was lucid enough to witness her own psychosis and several times, she turned to me and said, "Da Breo, I can't hold it together. I won't be able to see justice for my child". The apologetic rapist and his lawyer devised a twist, which was to say that Elusine had known of the sexual relationship between her child and her boyfriend and had allowed it, as it had gone on for so long in a one-room house.

In a final twist, due to Elusine's fully public declarations that she would kill this man if it were the last thing she ever did, and because a whole village had witnessed her slicing at him with her cutlass, she was charged with attempted murder. By the end of the fiasco, Elusine was declared incompetent to continue standing trial, the state authorities took the child from her, and everyone went "free", leaving us stunned by all of the wicked meanings of this word. Everyone walked free.

Elusine witnessed her victimhood acknowledged and then erased, leaving her with a second-order vulnerability caused by the law. One might call it an Iatrogenic disorder, which normally refers to an illness caused by medicine itself, but this time, it was an illness exacerbated by the law. She now avoided all humanity, realizing that they judged her demise to be a personal, psychological problem as though she were the sole author of her own suffering. There was no consideration of the worldly power relations that had brought her there.

One day following, as Elusine and I sat watching the setting sun burst into its usual flames and dragging jagged streaks of red through the blues of haunted skies, we wept, arms around each other.

"I am crying because my mind is broken", she said to me. "Why are you?"

"My heart", I replied.

She considered the ocean at our feet. "I thought that all the sad African women were at the bottom of that sea in the Atlantic", she mused. "Yet here we still are".

Sitting alone in her overgrown, weedy garden several moons later, bowls of holy water turned over and dry, Elusine took a knife and allowed the blood to run from her veins. More than a decade has passed, but whenever I drive past her village, I imagine I see her going by, long skirts sweeping the pitch, the trees above shaking out her laughter from amongst their leaves and branches. "Forget tea", she calls out to me, "Take a rum". Her laughter is like cowrie-shell bracelets dancing in the breeze. I want to ask her if, in her death, she at last feels free.

Chapter 9

The Counselor

Darkness falls upon me. The sun is overtaken by the infinite stars of the night sky, and it looks like a great galactic garden, a flower garden of stars. Nature blooms at night with planets instead of flowers, but what gets me is the vast blackness of this. It's all too much. Unlike the starry heavens, I want to lie low. I want to bury myself amongst the herbs and the fragrant earth. I have no potential.

The last client of yesterday told me she had been in the mental hospital several times in her life, all due to witchcraft. When she was 14, she said, a man forced his way into her mother's house and made her open her legs. She screamed, and she knew that all the neighbors heard her, but nobody came. He took off her panties, then took a big, long snake out of his pocket and sent it up inside her vagina. He told her, "This saarpent is a spirit under my control. I sent it up inside your body to live there, and I will control it. You will now do anything I say". The client told me that four children grew in her belly due to this witchcraft, but she has prayed steadfastly like her mother told her to do. She rebuked the satan. Now, at 64 years of age, the four children grown and gone, that saarpent has finally left her body and she has a little peace, despite the medications.

I looked at her and listened to her, and then I said the session was over. There is nothing I can do about this whole saarpent business and why should I. She is already old and over with it. So, I just listen. There is nothing to do.

Many clients are similar. They lost a house they want a house. They lost their job they want a job. Their husband beat them they want another one. What can I do? I am a counselor, but I have no counsel to give. I listen for an hour, then they go. They want me to be like them; that is what it is. They want to take me over. The lady with the saarpent, she kept saying about it over and over, hoping I could feel like if it was inside me too. But I shut her down in time. Bitch.

Over here is a mountain. It's not like other mountains where all the different shades and textures of green comfort and twist each other in a race to meet the sky. Not like the mountains that burp out some smoke from time to time and make us shiver below. No, this mountain is all dry, brown, and fossilized. It is a mountain of files I took home to work on last …. last …. Wait. What day is it? They are calling from the office to get the files, but I told my granny to say I don't dey.

DOI: 10.4324/9781003223603-11

My relationship failed. I had loved that boy; I really had. He saw me through my B.A. then he saw me through my M.A. He was the first one to be proud when I got my first job as a counselor. When I started working and told him that my book-learning had actually not prepared me for working with living people, he was the first to get scared and tell me to find a supervisor. I asked my employers for a supervisor, but they said there were none around here, nor any networks in the outer territories either. Only 15,000 people live on this island; no supervisor is among them. Yet, they keep sending us out to work with these clients who hack each other into pieces and bring Armageddon in their pockets like saarpents. I don't think they understand what we go through, getting eaten alive every day by issues. Abusers are cannibals. They don't eat the flesh but the lives of other people. While my bosses sit in their air-conditioned office. Bitches.

Where is the endorphin rush that front-line workers are supposed to feel? Where is the inherent goodness? I imagined that I would be full of altruistic purpose and compassion, but I'm not. At least I'm not as bad as my colleague in the office to the left who literally shouts at her clients. Literally insults them and shouts. I get it. Abusive husbands and cheating wives who call each other mudder cunt. Beaten and silenced children. They aren't nice. And the colleague to the right, like Mother Teresa, always a quiet voice. Bitch.

At night, I dream I see dripping red all about.

My sweet granny is at the door again, knocking, knocking. If I open it, I will see a shock in her eyes. My hair standing on ends like Medusa. My eyes blood red like Dracula because I saw night make morning yet again. Granny wants to give me those pills the doctor prescribed. Never mind, granny, my sweet granny, just let me sleep a little more. I'll go to work tomorrow. If they call me from the office, just tell them I don' dey, granny. Honestly. I don' dey.

Part II

Spirit Possession

Chapter 10

Vladimir

He roamed the forests and coastlines, bare-backed and bare-footed, machete in hand, crocus bag over a shoulder, dog at his heels. In the bag, he carried all he ever needed: a Swiss army knife given him by a soldier, a slingshot, and a piece of fishing line he'd liberated from an old sailor by the shore. By the age of ten, there was no species of flesh, fowl nor good red herring that Vladimir could not trap, shoot, skin, and cook, seasoning peppers plucked from whichever garden was handy. In his bag, he sometimes brought a hunt home to his family. The crowded, noisy household comprised brothers with whom he would violently spar, sisters he pitied, a harshly domineering father, and a mother that Vlad utterly despised. In other words, his home was a battleground of power struggles, but Vlad felt some satisfaction in sharing the hunt sometimes, simply because each member of the crowded house was a better cook than the other. Oil down, pepper pot, chutneys, and wild meat stews. The food they shared was their single commonality.

Vladimir also trapped education like he trapped prey. Dirty school house, half of a lead pencil, buttons missing from a frayed school shirt handed down an embarrassing number of times. But he kept his eyes on his teachers, and their words found fertile soil in his brain. Not that he engaged them at all; he was a non-participatory student; a silent and guarded boy. "You see how he is quiet, quiet?" one teacher mused. "Don't let that fool you. It's those still waters that drown you". Teachers did not discuss Vladimir much further than that, but they did wonder about the intensity with which he sharpened his lead pencils with that Swiss army knife he always carried. "That kid is a psychopath, hear what I'm telling you". Even as they graded him A in physics, A in anatomy, A in history, A in math, they muttered "You see his eyes? Like a fucking serpent. He'll petrify you. Freeze you to fucking death. Like a fucking psycho".

Three main events framed the trajectory of Vladimir's life and caused his personality to curve toward an evolution not indicated at his birth. In history books he read of a Romanian prince whose name he shared and whose military tactics fascinated him, particularly since the military stance defined the prince's personal ontology, his philosophy of life and his daily habits as well. Thus inspired by the prince, Vladimir began to stalk a new prey, his first human, selected as a follow up

DOI: 10.4324/9781003223603-13

to the first defining event of some years prior, his abuse by an elderly teacher. The planning was easy for Vlad.

Late one afternoon in his 16th year, Vladimir stepped out onto a mud path high up in the hills of seven colors, catching his old teacher on his routine trek home. "Remember me?" The teacher sized up the boy before him, five foot six or so, sun-burnished skin, unkempt *coco-piole* hair, and a long wooden pike in his hands. There was something about his eyes.

"I was two years old at the time", Vladimir told him in a voice hoarse like autumn leaves. "But I'm not two years old anymore". Recognition dawned too late in his teacher's eyes. It didn't take more than a minute for Vlad to have him flat on his belly in the mud, hog tied and eating dirt. Vlad pulled his long pike and jammed it into the teacher's anus, then with a small rock, he pounded it upward with slow, surgical precision, missing all of the vital organs that might offer a faster death until the tip of the pike protruded from teacher's shoulder. The teacher tried to scream many times during the hours it took him to finally die, but nothing came out except bubbling blood. Vladimir left both ends of the pike prominently visible so there could be no question about the intent of the procedure.

Meanwhile, and this was the third and most crucial turning point, Vladimir experienced the first full release of the rage he had nurtured in his soul from the age of two, his first orgasmic experience. Henceforth, blood became his eucharist, but deep within himself, Vlad simultaneously felt a deep void opening.

Franz Fanon wrote about the oppressed, colonial subject who eventually (but not always) becomes an oppressor. He describes how overlapping layers of tension, conflict, and disruption live on in abused children, as in subjugated societies. He wrote:

> The native is always on the alert ... he is overpowered but not tamed; he is treated as an inferior but he is not convinced of his inferiority. He is patiently waiting until the settler is off his guard to fly at him. The native's muscles are always tensed.
>
> (Fanon, 2002, p. 41)

No news reports accompanied the discovery of the corpse. No one finding it rotting and bloated, driven through from stem to stern with a razor-sharpened pike, could overcome their horror sufficiently to write, but rumors of a demonic being flying around the countryside began to spread. At first, they whispered that this could only be the workings of a maniac, but on further castigation, they pinned it on higher forces. "Only a demon could do this kind of a business". Nobody made any connection between this event and the silent, feral boy slipping through the forest with his equally silent dog. People were generally happier to place blame on supernatural entities.

People of the forest are wont to sleep, dream, and talk stories of the "other"; of energies that arise out of nature rather than a mother's womb. Indeed, to sleep on a bed of damp and pungent foliage while invisible beings croak, hiss, and rustle at each other in the dark leaves forest dwellers with no shadow of a doubt of the existence of the unknown, unseen. On the other hand, others passing through might well name the forest psychotic in its own right. Things are heard but not seen, felt but not revealed, acting upon you and holding you in a grip that you can neither name nor escape. This condition is not strange to people of the deep woods, but admittedly, some find it terrifying in its realness. These "people" include psychologists who, if westernized thoroughly enough, will dismiss and deride notions of the unconscious and emotionally bludgeon both nature and humankind into submission with good, tidy scientific explanations and behaviors. On the other hand, when cultures embrace their dark spaces, psychological work becomes infinitely more clear, even as it shows itself to be complex and fearful in real terms.

Fanon wrote of the inherent affinity for myth and magic that accompanies natives of the rainforest or of the global south.

> Terrifying myths … are so frequently found in underdeveloped communities. These are maleficent spirits which intervene every time a step is taken in the wrong direction. . a whole series of tiny animals or giants which create around the native a world of prohibitions far more terrifying that the world of the settler. This atmosphere of myth and magic frightens me.
>
> Fanon, 2002, p. 43)

Fanon himself saying that he was terrified by tales of magical beings and the supernatural grants us free passage to also confess, as doctors, psychiatrists, or counselors, of this apprehension within ourselves. But we have all taken our vows, and in my view, we are no more free to turn away from open – heart surgery in an operating theatre because of personal queasiness than we are free to turn away from the open-soul transactions that occur, according to Fanon, on the phantasmic plane.

Take Haiti as an example where sexual abuse can be so beyond the pale of one's tender imagination that only subscription to the supernatural will do.

> In the fairy tales, the *Tonton Macoute* was a bogeyman, a scarecrow with human flesh. He wore denim overalls and carried a knapsack made of straw. In his knapsack, he always had scraps of naughty children, whom he dismembered to eat as a snack…. Outside the fairy tales, they roamed the streets in broad daylight … My father might have been a *Macoute*. He was a stranger who, when my mother was eighteen years old, grabbed her on her way back from school. He dragged her into the cane fields, and pinned her down on the ground. …. He kept pounding her until she was too stunned to make a sound. When he was done, he made her keep her face in the dirt, threatening to shoot her if she looked up. For months she was afraid that he would creep out of the night and kill her in her sleep. She was terrified that he would come and tear out the child growing inside her. At night, she tore her sheets and bit off pieces of her own flesh when she had nightmares.
>
> (Danticat, 2015, pp. 137–138)

Wotan

Turning to an archetype that Jung has used to describe oppressed individuals who not only turn to singular acts of personal revenge but, when working in groups, they can turn to military acts of global destruction, mowing down material infrastructure and whole ecosystems as well as the humans in their path. This is Wotan. In his darkest guise, Wotan the wanderer is the ancient god of storm and frenzy. He lusts after revenge and the complete annihilation wrought by war, observing no boundaries or restraints. Worse, he is immanently capable of luring masses of accomplices, enablers, and allies to work alongside him, committing unimaginable acts of terror. Connected to the figure of Dionysus, who also is a restless wanderer who works magic and creates unrest, Wotan is often depicted as a ghostly hunter leading his retinue and "flickering like a will o' the wisp through the storm night" (Sjöstedt-Hughes, 2023).

Back to Vladimir, it was decades after his first taste of blood; after his prowess as pilot of fighter aircraft in the military had earned him several medals for unusual fearlessness and bravery in the face of apocalyptic reality, that Vlad entered medical school qualifying first as a surgeon of uncanny precision and then as a psychiatrist. With his inherent resentment toward people in power and a determination never to fall under the control of anyone, Vlad rose to the top of any field he entered. Like his Kalinago ancestors before him, he preferred to fight, flee or die rather than subject himself to any authority, but it was acknowledged by colleagues and superiors that he had now become equally as adept at saving lives as a doctor, as he had been at destroying them when he was a soldier. When Vlad read of psychosis for the first time he had a flush of recognition. He knew that he had experienced psychosis many times in his life beginning in childhood, and that he had inadvertently, intuitively, individuated himself out of them. Frankl refers to this as "self-transcendence", and as Maslow wrote, the "will to meaning", man's primary concern, is even available to infants (Maslow, 1969, quoted in Frankl, 2000, p. 86). During his period of study in psychiatry, battling Post Traumatic Stress Disorder (PTSD) both from his military service and from child sexual abuse, Vladimir entered the process of psychoanalytic psychotherapy, faced the humbling task of confronting the evil that he had encouraged to fester deep within his personal shadow, and he began to heal. Luckily, he found an analyst who was not sidetracked by the idea of psychology as an abstract elitist philosophy, but who understood its application to victims of torture and war, both of the organized military and of the individually wounded kind.

Vladimir now learned to hold his gaze upon the tensions of his opposites without fear. Like Jung's image of the Ouroboros (Jung, CW 954/968, p. 78), in which opposites face each other in conscious awareness, Vladimir could hold the duality of the extreme pain of his childhood victimhood and his own capacity for extreme violence alongside a powerfully emerging gift for healing. He learned to perceive himself not as disjointed but as unified and whole. As he began to discern these diverse parts with clarity, Vlad also recognized that he was no longer the same; that an alchemical process of transformation had been initiated, and he was standing on the threshold of deep change. It is one of the tenets of Jungian psychology that what poisons you also can heal you. As both Jung and von Franz described, this type of journey marks the alchemical trail between the latent Self and the manifest Self, but it is not for those without courage. Vladimir finally "looked in the Schopenhauerian mirror, in which the unconscious becomes aware of its own face" (Jung, CW 14, 129).

This attainment of consciousness is the goal of psychotherapy, or as Jung would say, "the supreme aim of the *opus psychologicum*" (Jung, 944/968, p. 26). Vlad could not give anyone a vow of consistent, linear forward movement, but he was intensely curious and committed to reducing the arbitrariness with which he had swerved from ecstasy to despair in the past. Thus, with the metaphorical philosopher's stone firmly in grasp, he walked steadily away from victimhood as an abused and tormented child; away from a destiny as *puer aeternus*, and toward rejuvenation and his Magnum Opus as a doctor of souls as well as bodies.

In Jungian psychology, as Stein wrote, "The first duty of the ethically minded person is to become as conscious as possible of his own shadow" (Stein, 1995, p. 17). Jung wrote, "The shadow is a moral problem that challenges the whole ego-personality, for no one can become conscious of the shadow without considerable moral effort" (CW, vol. 9ii, para 14).

Vladimir was in his late fifties before being able to address the sex abuse trauma that had befallen him at age two and had continued for years. When he learned how to assimilate his shattered ego, he became good, but meanwhile, as Junot Diaz wrote of his own childhood sexual abuse:

> That shit cracked the planet of me in half, threw me completely out of orbit, into the lightless regions of space where life is not possible. I can say, truly, que casi me destruyo.
>
> (Díaz, 2018)

Emotional awareness is necessary for depth psychological work and transformation and Vladimir, despite (or because of) everything he had been through, was wide open to change. Though he could not have planned it in advance, Vlad learned to be a healer as part of being cured from a deep affliction. Like Dante he literally lost himself in the dark woods and escaped his inferno only after reaching the lowermost point of despair. Without human guide, he put himself through the cycle of affliction, salvation and transformation which is a cycle as old as our planet and available to Everyman, though it usually calls for a skilled and fearless guide or a therapist.

In psychotherapy, as Vladimir's entangled constellation of emotional issues began to unfold, one of the issues that he was able to articulate was an old Father Wound. Vladimir allowed himself to pull it into awareness as he realized that the ancient father wound continued to impair his ability to have successful intimate relationships in the current day.

The Father Wound in Men

The father wound in men renders them very easily offended and intolerant of others' emotions. People in close relationships with Vlad felt they had to walk on eggshells around him so as not to cause him more distress than he was evidently carrying, and they would consequently themselves feel emotionally neglected both in terms of self-neglect and in terms of neglect by their partner, Vlad. If Vladimir had had children, he would have perpetuated this emotionally neglected feeling down to them, and this is how the cycle becomes intergenerational. In this text, Yusuf and Nile also suffered from severe father wounds, making their childhood traumas all the more complex – Yusuf as orphan and then sexually abused by the state system; Nile as abused and then abandoned in multiple ways. In cultures where men father and then abandon their sons, a father wound is predictable in all varying degrees of severity.

The father complex includes more than the birth father but other male parental or authority figures as well. In terms of a full cultural complex, the whole patriarchy can be implicated for its totalitarian dominance and oppression on the one hand, and silence in the face of physical and mental torture of its citizens on the other. Cultural and gender norms inform this as well, and clearly, as we collectively watch what is happening between Israel and Gaza in this moment of my writing, we see the same principle playing out politically, writ large.

For Vlad, the little boy in him that had been crushed by an overbearing and abusive father and later violated by a man he looked up to as a father, was left feeling chronically "not good enough" to warrant the love, respect, and protection that ought to come from a Dad. Jungians believe that children are born wired for relationships and are able to recognize masculinity as well as femininity from infancy. The kind of masculinity that one is exposed to from infancy sculpts one's expectations of life.

Jung wrote copiously about his own Father Wound. His father was not abusive, but as an adolescent Jung observed him be passive with no spiritual backbone; ground; a pastor with no faith. Unable to engage with him on the heated passions that fueled Jung's interests in psychology, spirituality, and world views, Jung wrote that he dearly missed having a father who would show pride in him and save him from the hollowness that he felt in his home. Jung's relationship with Freud, a well-known father-son dynamic, not only sculpted the direction of Jung's life following their meeting, but was potent enough to transform the direction of the disciplines of psychology and psychiatry as well.

Vladimir became a soldier at war, and war is a military manifestation of fatherhood in which soldiers and sufferers of PTSD are forced to live the narrative of the "fatherland". We see this playing out today, as the image and likeness of some historic fatherlands appear to be manifesting, like the *Babadook*, as monstrous, cunning, and demoniacal.

Like other boys in his position, Vladimir projected the hurt feelings of the father wound outward by cheating on his women and not trusting in any respect offered by other men even when it was genuine. He kept a defensive guard up at all times, preferring to accumulate material gains so he could quantify a sense of worthiness.

Inner Child Healing

The father wound manifests in various conditions, such as if a father makes you afraid in his presence, or if a father is so passive that he does not protect you from an overly domineering mother. A father wound may be a conceptual attack or perceived abandonment, or a combination of real and conceptual experiences.

This is only one part of the enmeshment of psychic turmoil that held Vladimir in its grip for the better part of his life, considering that the culture in which he was raised, the Latin American and Caribbean Region, comprises levels of violence that are listed as among the highest in the world. According to the World Population Review, 2023, Venezuela, Trinidad and Tobago, Guyana, Brazil, El Salvador, Honduras, and Jamaica are in the top ten most violent places on earth (World Population Review.com, 2023).

In Jungian scholarship, the father archetype is associated with kingship, gods, authority, and order. It is a powerful archetype that becomes an equally powerful negative complex if fathers are experienced as absent, passive, and emotionally unavailable on the one hand and critical, blaming, or abusive on the other. Even Jung, who enjoyed his father-son relationship with Freud for some time, suffered years of emotional turmoil when the relationship ended.

In therapy, if clients are able to face this wound and heal it, an incredible storehouse of energy may be released for living more creatively and consciously, as in Vladimir's case of going on to significant professional and personal success.

Jungian psychology speaks of transformation, redemption, and the alchemy of self-reflection as the work of a lifetime.

> Reflection should be understood not simply as an act of thought, but rather as an attitude. It is a privilege born of human freedom in contradistinction to the compulsion of natural law. As the word itself testifies (reflection means literally "bending back"), reflection is a spiritual act that runs counter to the natural process; as an act whereby we stop, call something to mind, form a picture, and take up a relation to and come to terms with what we have seen. It should therefore be understood as an act of becoming conscious.
>
> (Jung, Collected Works, vol. 11, para 235 n.)

Dionysus

Although Vladimir did not learn how to describe the archetypal energies that had arisen to save him on his journey of individuation until he underwent analysis in his middle age, he later understood the transformative power of Dionysus, the god of excessive sexual revelry, wine, and the essential lifeblood of nature. Called Dionysus by the Greeks, he is known as Osiris in Egypt and as Acan in the ancient Mayan kingdom. To the Romans, he is known as Bacchus, god of the Bacchanal, a concept which in contemporary times has become quintessentially Caribbean.

Bacchus is the mythical god of wine-making, orchards, fertility, festivity, insanity, ritual madness, and religious ecstasy. Born of Zeus and Semele, Bacchus is known for the ritual frenzy that he would induce. As Dionysus Eleutherios, The Liberator, his music and ecstatic dance freed his followers from self-conscious fear and subverted the oppressive restraints of political power.

In a unique, historical manifestation of this archetype, Dionysus may be found alive in the land where 100,000 Jab-Jabs take the road at carnival time, in Jab Nation, Grenada. The term "Jab" derives from the French word "Diable", which Caribbeans doubled up for good measure. Jab-Jab in effect means a Double Devil.

Jabs paint themselves blacker than black, losing themselves in the midnight from which they emerge, drums blazing, at Jouvay, which derives from the French "Jour Overt" or the opening of the day. Using black paint, old oil, molasses or tar, the primary idea of Jab is Blackness. Blackness is resistance. It is such an underworld decent that the only way upward at the end of the journey is by explosive rebirth.

Jab-Jab is a full assault on reality. If the definition of *taste* in a class culture may be understood by Bourdieu's description, "taste is an incorporated principle of classification which governs all forms of incorporation ... the body is the most indisputable materialization of class taste" (Bourdieu, 1987, p. 210), then to be black, sensual, entranced and incontrovertibly in command is therefore a most manifest upset of the status quo in colonized society.

The Jab-Jab archetype arises from the collective unconscious. In the Caribbean, it differentiates into an archetype of its own strongly feeling-toned culture, related to the theme of slavery, colonialism, and modern-day patriarchy. It relates to a foundational psychological need; to put down the Apollonian constraints of the quotidian and resist oppression in all of its formats. The Jab is a living archetypal symbol of rebellion.

In the Caribbean's colorist, classicist culture, some Caribbeans take Jab as the quintessential shadow. Immoral, hyper-sensualized, and anarchist, the Jab is at once alluring and feared. This confluence of racial and sexual complexes carries overwhelming psychic energy and archetypal meaning.

Even in Rome during their Liberalia festivals, the state regarded the bacchanal as subversive because in them, classes, genders, and races mixed freely and transgressed social and moral constraints.

Fanon described the bacchanal this way:

The circle of the dance is a permissive circle. It protects and permits. At certain times on certain days, men and women come together at a given place and there, under the solemn eye of the tribe, fling themselves into a seemingly unorganized ... ecstatic dance.

(Fanon, 2002,, p. 44)

No person would manifest Dionysus more fiercely than Vladimir. A violated, abused, and angry boy who had wandered the forests throughout childhood and adolescence, living on what he hunted until he began to hunt human prey. Dripping poison from one hand, so to speak, and honey from the other, Vladimir was savage and salvation in one entity.

Dionysus' traditional scepter, his *thyrsus*, is historically wound with ivy and dripping with honey, both a wand and a weapon used to destroy those who oppose freedom. In Dionysus' Caribbean context, Grenada's Jabs similarly carry the traditional *thyrsus*, but theirs are wound with poison ivy and drip with live serpents, representing a clear and present danger yet simultaneously calling on followers to accept possession and empowerment at the behest of the gods of music and dance themselves. Also known as the god of theater, in no place has Dionysus' archetypal energy found a more fertile and fitting personification than in the Jab Nation.

One of the most insidious poisons of the colonialism project was to separate Indigenous people from their own unifying principles, for example, that we are Caribbean. Instead, we were cut into differentiated colors, shades of colors, and tones of shades, not in the interest of diversity but to foist racism upon us until we learned to be racist with each other; to separate, measure, categorize, and label like diseases in the Diagnostic Statistical Manual (DSM). But Jab is the equalizer. Jab is either black or blacker and in this we are all equal and free.

Dr. Peter Sjostedt-Hughes describes how archetypal energy can manifest or possess not only in a single human being, but whole nations at a time. Take Wotan, who creates roving unrest and stirs up strife, he exudes energy potent enough to wake up like an extinct volcano in countries that are so-called civilized, "armed with rucksack and lute", or as the Yemeni resistance has recently been described, "with Nikes and flip flops". On the other side of the coin, as Sjostedt-Hughes wrote, Wotan is recognized in the hundreds of thousands of youth who marched for Hitler, literally bringing the whole of Germany to its feet. In a great irony, Wotan can also be seen in the waning numbers of disillusioned soldiers who are currently marching for Israel to complete the genocide of Palestinians in Gaza. As I currently write from a so-called civilized place where children are nevertheless abused at a rate of one in three (Jones et al.), I shiver in my shoes to wonder what this implies for their futures; for the futures of all the world's children. We know very much about victims, but we have very little research and very few statistics and descriptors of perpetrators. However, they will surely count among the numbers of mentally ill individuals whose minds break under the weight of the harm that they cause and the harm that was caused to them.

To say that I see Wotan in numerous male clients who have been abused as children and have grown up volcanically violent as a result, I have no hesitation in ascribing this energy to cultures where CSA is normalized, along with the silence and complicity of bystanders. Child Abuse Psychosis, the diagnostic term that I propose for breakdowns brought about by childhood sexual abuse, often has violence as a significant part of its symptom list. As Sjostedt-Hughes writes, Wotan is the god of intoxication and exuberance, the unleasher of passions, and the lust of battle. Linked with Dionysus, Wotan shakes up societies, states, military units and psychic bodies, acting on the high pressure of so-called civilization and blowing it away.

Victims of Violence and Introvert Homes

Vladimir became a wealthy man. Worldly, accomplished and highly respected, his distrust of other people nevertheless increased with age. He designed and built his own house, perched on the top of a cliff with perilous drops to the ocean on three sides and a tall gate on the forth. When I visited, I was struck by the similarity with Elusine's property, though hers existed on a different island, and at the furthest end of material capacity from his. Vladimir had a swimming pool that butted up against high courtyard walls so you could not climb out on the far side; there was one way in and one way back out. Several flights of stone stairs lead nowhere, which one would only discover having climbed them to the summit. Corridors became increasingly narrow so that at the end, only cats and spirits could pass through; human guests would need to turn around and come back. Vladimir's social anxiety remained acute throughout his lifespan. While he was able enough to go out in the days and work relentlessly at his vocation, becoming known as a highly skilled neurologist and healer, in the evenings, he retreated to his introvert house, relaxed and happy to be alone; silent dogs at his bedside.

References

Bourdieu, P. (1987) *Distinction: A Social Critique of the Judgement of Taste*, Published March 12, 2010 by Routledge

Danticat, E. (2015). *Breath, Eyes, Memory*. Soho Press, Inc.

Díaz, J. (2018, April 9). The silence: the legacy of childhood trauma. *The New Yorker*. https://www.newyorker.com/magazine/2018/04/16/the-silence-the-legacy-of-childhood-trauma

Fanon, F. (2002) *Wretched of the Earth*. Penguin, 1st edition (originally published 1961).

Frankl, V. (2000). *Man's Search for Ultimate Meaning*. Perseus Publishing.

Sjöstedt-Hughes, P. (2023, September 10). *C. G. Jung – Essay on Wotan*. Dr Peter Sjöstedt-Hughes: Philosopher of Mind and Metaphysics. https://www.philosopher.eu/others-writings/essay-on-wotan-w-nietzsche-c-g-jung/

Stein, M. (1995). *Encountering Jung on Evil*. Princeton University Press.

Chapter 11

Yara

The Transcendent

"Where is my light?" He called up at her window. "Where is the light that comes from the hills?"

Yara heard her Daddy's voice and flew across the room to the second-floor window, where she pushed the shutters open to reveal his laughing face in the courtyard below.

"There she is! The light that comes from beside the sea!" Ignatio stretched his arms upwards, and Yara barely restrained herself from jumping out of the window toward him. She leapt down the stairs in one, and in two, she was engulfed in her father's embrace. "Daddy! You took so long!"

Yara's father was a forest ranger of some kind, if she understood it correctly, and he covered a vast territory. He went around the hills and rivers of Guatemala with other colleagues, preserving nature and animals, cleaning up the mangroves, protecting the forests from illegal logging, and catching thieves who came in the night for jade. From the fierce whispers between her parents in their room, Yara deduced that his work often put him in danger from other people, and his wife lived in fear and resentment that one day he would not return. But return, he always did, spilling gifts from his pockets for his woman and their only child. Always gifts, never money. "Daddy is like weather", Yara thought. "He comes like storms and leaves like ebbing tide".

"Look at all this wealth!" Ignatio would say to his wife, Conception, sweeping his arms at the mountains in the distance. "Who is rich like us?"

"I can't cook the hills", his wife would reply. "I can't buy groceries with moonlight!"

Yara saw her father frown during conversations like these. "But you can!" he told her mother. "Don't you understand that without this we'd be nothing?" Realizing that Yara was listening intently, he would manifest a smile that went from ear to ear, from mountain to shore.

"Besides, where would Yara swim, if I did not preserve her rivers? We have 18 of them and each one of them belongs to her. They are her birthright. The most sacred work I could possibly do is ensure that those rivers keep running for our child".

But Conception shot back, "Do you really think it is *you* that keeps the rivers of Guatemala running? And you call that sacred work? I cannot feed my family on the sacred, Ignatio!" she said, real bitterness in her tone.

DOI: 10.4324/9781003223603-14

Ignatio stayed quiet for a moment. Yara held her breath. She felt that he was very angry and trying to control it. "You are very beautiful", he eventually said to his wife. "But something is missing. I think you are missing a heart".

Ignatio spent many evenings when he was at home, sitting on the grass in the field behind the house, back against a tree, guitar in hand. A modern-day Orpheus, Ignatio sang in a deep baritone and with profound emotion, and neighbors would come from all around to sit and join him in chorus, some bringing other instruments to play.

Leaving formal book learning to others better suited, Ignatio trained his daughter in the contemplative arts, reminding her often, "Keep an eye on your heart. Your heart holds many secrets that it will take you the rest of your life to discover. Once you unlock them, the universe will follow". For years, he did his best to cajole Yara into learning his guitar as well, or his flute, but she declined, preferring instead to lie on her back in the tall grass and listen to her father play.

In the days and years to come, Yara would remember one particular verse from a song her father sang; one that was especially popular with the villagers. As they sang it with such fervor, each and every time they met, Bahira wondered if there was any significance to their mention of Guerrilleros and their manner of vanishing among the people as they marched untouched through Guatemala's forests.

Ignatio had been gone this time for many moons, but Yara shouted at her mother, blocked her ears and ran away hard when it was suggested to her that this time, he would not return. Just as the sky began to purple one dusky evening, somewhere deep within the earth's crust two massive plates started grinding against each other and way up above on Yara's street, there came an eerie sound of creaking. The ground rolled and villagers stumbled in their tracks. Taking stock of the situation they raised the alarm "Earthquake!" and pandemonium ensued. Yara felt the earth's tremors right through her body but did not register the sense of fear that seized the rest of her community. She wondered where her father might be on a night such as this and she turned in the direction of her mother's house. That is when she heard her father's voice, as clearly as if he was whispering directly into her ear. "Pay attention!", he said urgently, and that whisper was more compelling than the shifting of the earth under Yara's feet.

She peered into the fast descending darkness where villagers ran helter-skelter through the narrow streets, some shouting for their children and others, for no reason that Yara could determine, beginning to heave stones through shop windows, breaking glass. Through the madness, Yara saw three men coming toward her, gesticulating in her direction, eyes fixed, strides purposeful. This time, Yara felt a sudden rush of intense fear and when her father's voice called her name again, she turned and sped on winged feet in the opposite direction turning only to confirm that yes, there they came running after her and she recognized the look of hunters tracking prey. Chaos lay behind and beneath Yara, and the blackness of night had completely dropped, but she ran for her life, blindly pushing through the dense under bush and following only one sound, that of Ignatio's Orphic direction. "Run to the river".

The water was pitch cold as Yara slid herself quietly in and it moved with more urgency than she had ever experienced before. Wading into the tangle of mangroves, Yara felt herself lifted horizontally by the rushing current, river rocks and loosened debris slapping and pounding into her body. But Yara was safe and she held on silently, losing sense of how many hours passed as she floated there, wedged in among the roots. The night was wicked with rain. Wind whistled in sudden ferocious bursts and then just as suddenly died away. "Don't be afraid", whispered her father's voice. "Hide yourself in the blue. Your father is here". At last Yara understood where her father had gone all this time. He had transmigrated into the weather and would always, always protect her from there.

It was daybreak before Yara allowed herself to rise from the water, accompanied by howler monkeys screeching the sun back into the sky. It was a brilliant dawn, a day so clear the very ends of the earth could be seen, but it took Yara a very long time to hike back home. She had run a much longer distance than she remembered, and by the time she approached her village everything had changed. Many of the homes and shops had collapsed and heaps of rubble were piled up everywhere, but on her street, most buildings remained standing, and men and women rushed around putting things upright again, sweeping dust and debris off the road and chattering with each other about the near catastrophe. Most distracting for Yara, however, was the sight of the three men who had chased her leaning up on the side of her mother's house, casually chatting and in fact it was they who touched her mother's arm and gesticulated with their chins in Yara's direction.

"Where were you?!" Her mother hurried to her side. "Where were you?!" but Yara instantly felt that something was off; something more than the shaking earth and the weeping skies. She looked into her mother's face, saw no worry there and carefully gauged her words before responding. "I was with my father", she said.

"What?" Her mother put her palm to Yara's brow, as though checking for a fever. "Are you alright? Where *were* you?" Yara saw that the three men were listening to what she would reply.

"With my father", she said again. "We were in the blue".

Several women from the surrounding houses had gathered around by this, having realized that Yara went missing in the confusion of the night. They took her by the shoulders, looked deeply into her eyes, checked her head for injuries and tut-tutted among themselves. But Yara gave the same answers as before. "I was with my father. We were in the weather".

In the days that followed, as Yara followed instructions shouted at her by any of the village aunties to take up laundry, run to the shop, help babysit at the community center, and so forth, Yara had a sense of being perpetually stalked. She could be seen holding her head at a strange angle, listening out for something she would not explain, and at least three more times before her mother managed to pack up and leave that village, Yara felt it necessary to run for her life again, neighborhood men on her heels, while she followed her father's voice. "Run to the green, Yara, hurry!".

She never failed to return, sometimes days later, finding her mother strangely unconcerned. Yara never came to any harm because, as she heard villagers whisper, she could shift into the wind, like her father. The child had lost her mind and learned to do very strange things. So had her mother, apparently, because as soon as communications were reestablished in the village and in their house, Mother began to spend most of the day talking on various computer applications, with men, in very intimate tones. Often she took selfies with Yara, posting them online with big smiles and gay-looking postures, while Yara remained dissociated, hyper alert, and tilting her head toward the distant mountain breeze.

It took several months for Yara and her mother to travel northward to Toronto, where one of the men Yara recognized from the computer was waiting to help them off the Greyhound. In a daze of time, grief, dislocation and fear, Yara settled into a condominium with her mother and the new "husband", started a new school where she gave every appearance of being very well adjusted and acclimatized, and allowed herself to be "looked after" by this new attentive man.

One evening, after Yara had not managed to finish the full cup of sweet coco-tea that was always made for her at dinner, she excused herself early and went to bed, feeling somewhat nauseous. She awoke hours later when all was dark and quiet, and she felt drops of water fall into her face. Struggling for consciousness, Yara could not break the hold that a deep sleep had on her, but the searing pain in her belly forced her to try. She pushed and twisted, fighting an unbearable knifing pain between her legs and realized that the water falling into her face was sweat from the stepfather's brow as he lay above her, breathing hard. Yara managed to turn her head away, facing the door and calling out as loudly as she could though her thoughts were cotton wool, "I'm not okay. Something's wrong".

Her mother stood in the doorway, watching quietly and not coming to her aid. The stepfather moved faster on Yara's bones and in a flash she understood. She had been trafficked to this man to earn their entry into this city, and to afford her mother the life style she always coveted but could never afford with such a man as Ignatio. Yara shook her head to clear it and another reality struck; she was drugged. And she knew that this then, was the common nightly routine into which she had been sold, all of her morning sluggishness and deep belly pains making every sense now. Yara called out from the depths of her soul, "Daddy!" and swiftly, her father came to her side with more clarity than he ever had before.

"They are taking all the beauty out", Yara heard him say. "Now cultivate the hatred you have never felt but which you have inside you. It is better to explode yourself than surrender to this".

Yara reached way down into her blues and greens. She reached for her father's guitar, his flute, his voice in the wind, and the strength in his legs as they ran together through the forests of Guatemala.

To say that Yara screamed would not begin to describe the sound that came out of her body now. Rather, it was as though all of the hounds of hell set to barking at once; all of the hurricanes of the Pacific coast swirled up in one mighty wind; as though Zeus himself was hurling thunderbolts from end to end of that room; the sky blazed with the fires of Nyx.

In Greek mythology, Nyx is the goddess of the night. She is a primordial force, born of Chaos even before the dawn and the light of creation. Also called by the name of Night, or Nox in Rome, Nyx is most often depicted as dressed in black robes as she rides a horse-drawn chariot through the skies. In some Orphic accounts, Nyx is the mother of the stars and by other accounts she lives at the entrance to the underworld, having a terrifying nature. She is hard to identify, however, as Nyx also has the attribute of air, and cannot be held or seen.

When Dr. Andrade and I began to work with Yara, her mother, and her stepfather, it took us some time to recognize that the parents were both involved in trying to keep her drugged, silenced, and in the service of the man who had paid good money for perpetual access to this girl. Somehow, they determined that they could both fool the two of us, enlisting our assistance in making the child behave and psychologizing her into a state of gratefulness, hopelessness, and servitude. But Andrade being him and me being me, we both encouraged and relied upon Yara's connection to her birth father and the energies of the dark feminine that arose from the collective unconscious to save Yara's sanity and her life.

Since then, we have both recognized the archetypal energy of Nyx in numerous girl victims of child abuse psychosis. While the rage they express, if they can, is seen as unfeminine, uncivilized, insane and demonic, it is often precisely the force that they need in order to escape oppressions that are usually intergenerational, systematic and exceedingly difficult to exit on one's own. The energy personified by Nyx is there to be helpful and healing, thereafter to be integrated into the daily functioning of a healthy, peaceful, lifestyle, if possible. According to Kaballah we each have a lion within us, an *Aryeh* which represents courage, inner strength and discipline. And as Allen wrote "Black women need to see the importance of using their enraged voices because an enraged voice used to defend one's human rights is an act of intervention" (Allen, p. 33).

> "I can't be chained. I can't be a slave.
> I must go mad and go wild and get free"
> The Paw, Destan.

Child Trafficking

Unfolding before our eyes is a world crisis of epic proportions in which children are placed at great vulnerability and risk. In Syria today, more than 14 million people have been displaced, 5.8 million of which are children. In 2016, UNICEF (United Nations Children's Fund) reported that 306,000 Syrian children had been born as refugees since 2011, "their lives shaped by loss, deprivation, violence and fear". Child labor exploitation has become a widely established phenomenon (Kaya, 2020; Simsek, 2020) among refugees who have settled in Turkey, a "safe third country" (Haferlach & Kurban, 2017, p. 86). This multi-layered problem includes a lack of social protection mechanisms and obstacles to education (Akin, 2009. Turkish data declares that child labor and its attendant social issues have been a problem long before Syrian refugees arrived there (Lordoglu & Aslan, 2019).

Along with Syria, Greece has seen an unprecedented number of new refugee arrivals since 2016, plus others just passing through (Kitsantonis, 2019) and incidentally, Doctors Without Borders had only 20 field psychologists working with approximately 53,000 refugees in Greece at that time.

Without counting the numbers of children recently genocided in Gaza, and the multitudes more who have had their limbs blown off, there are currently more than 50 million children on the move around the world today, seeking a chance for a better life. While many of them may find good opportunities, leaving their homes puts all children at an increased risk of neglect, violence, and economic and sexual violence (UNICEF, 2016).

> Another problem is that many of those needing treatment have failed to come forward. Even if you have suffered abuse … that momentum to keep moving (is) still there … mental health … is not a priority for a population … struggling to survive.
> (Dedman, 2016, quoted in Khan, 2019. Apa.org./international/ global-insights/refugee-children-challenge)

While rates of poor mental health among populations of refugee children increase, they have little or no access to psychiatric healthcare due to "a lack of awareness regarding the availability of services, worries about discrimination in services, difficulties in communication because of language differences, and views of parents or relatives about the Western diagnostic paradigms" (Barghadoud et al., 2006). However, it is often from this very population that the most astute and capable healers and psychologists emerge, knowing firsthand the unique mental health challenges faced by their own kind. Indeed, as some of them become international educators, they urge that the conflicts and crises of the outer world are signals to mankind to awaken.

Human trafficking is a global issue not isolated to countries where there is civil or military unrest, to impoverished, third-world countries or to small island states that have easy access to the sea. In the 2022 Global Report on Trafficking in Persons (GLOTIP; UNODC, 2023), 53,800 cases of reported victims of trafficking were identified across 166 counties.

Statistics on human trafficking include cases of sexual exploitation, forced labor, and to a lesser degree forced marriage, illegal adoption, begging, and criminal activities.

Risk factors linked to an increased likelihood of victimization often correspond with a history of maltreatment or co-occurrence of different types of maltreatment (Meinck et al., 2021) and children who have experienced abuse, abandonment, or neglect, such as those in the child welfare system, are more likely to be targeted and victimized by traffickers (Reid et al., 2017; Latzman & Gibbs, 2020).

As we have noted several times in this text, the profession of psychology needs to expand itself to keep abreast of the many diverse manifestations of traumas manifesting in the world, and the interventions that would best offer healing to these individuals and groups.

References

Akin, L. (2009). Working conditions of the child worker in Turkish labour law. *Employee Responsibilities and Rights Journal*, *21*, 53–67. https://doi.org/10.1007/s10672-008-9098-7

Dedman, 2016, quoted in Khan, 2019. Apa.org./international/global-insights/refugee-children-challenge

Haferlach, L., & Kurban, D. (2017). Lessons learnt from the EU-Turkey refugee agreement in guiding EU migration partnerships with origin and transit countries. *Global Policy*, *8*, 85–93. https://doi.org/10.1111/1758-5899.12432

Kaya, A. (2020). Global migration: Consequences and responses working paper. Reception: Country report. https://doi.org/10.5281/zenodo.3665809

Kitsantonis, N. (2019). Rumors of open border prompt migrant protests in Greece. *The New York Times*. https://www.nytimes.com/2019/04/05/world/europe/greece-migrantprotest.html#:~:text="This%20is%20false%20information%2C%20the,and%20cross%2C"%20he%20added

Lordoglu, K., & Aslan, M. (2019). The invisible working force of minor immigrants: The case of Syrian children in Turkey. In G. Yılmaz, İ D. Karatepe, & T. Tören (Eds.), *Integration Through Exploitation: Syrians in Turkey* (pp. 55–66). Rainer Hampp Verlag.

Simsek, D. (2020). Integration processes of Syrian refugees in Turkey: 'Class-based integration'. *Journal of Refugee Studies*, *33*(3), 537–554. https://doi.org/10.1093/jrs/fey057

United Nations Children's Fund [UNICEF]. 2016, September 6). Uprooted: The growing crisis for refugee and migrant children. https://data.unicef.org/resources/uprooted-growing-crisis-refugee-migrant-children/

Part III

Rise of the Dark Feminine

Chapter 12

Bahira

To Kensington Market and its environs, all of the sound-makers in Toronto gathered sooner or later. Toronto is the cultural capital of Canada, and Kensington Market, bordered by College, Dundas, Spadina, and Bathurst streets, is not only Toronto's most vibrantly diverse neighborhood but a designated national historical site. First populated by Irish and Scottish immigrant laborers in the 1880s, Kensington soon became home to Italians and Eastern European Jews. By the 1930s, over 30 synagogues had sprung up alongside the original Victorian row houses, and successive waves of immigration continued to bring people from the Azores, the Caribbean, Portugal, China, Ethiopia, and several parts of Latin and South America. Over the years, an immense variety of groceries, cafes, and entertainment spots representing all of these cultures have planted their roots, bringing the fragrance and sounds of foreign shores to peaceful, explosive resonance in just this one place. With the Toronto Western Hospital, the Kensington Community Square, and the infamous Bellevue Park also there, each day dawns upon an eclectic mix of musicians, writers, jewelers, vintners and such, crisscrossing each other as they bustle through the narrow, pedestrian-filled streets. The 2016 census counted 17,945 residents and listed Chinese as the largest population, but there also are plenty of Rastafari with their distinctive accents, aromas, and beats. As for tourists, Kensington is crowded year round with visitors from everywhere, all of them feeling instantly at home in the living streets of the Market.

Around 2003, I undertook an internship at the Zen Buddhist Temple Toronto, which was located on College at Spadina back then, just on the outskirts of Kensington. One of my primary tasks was the ringing of the Evening Bell in the huge (cold) meditation hall and it proved one of the most challenging assignments that I have ever undertaken. Along with the Venerable Samu Sunim, there were two monks assigned to my personal education in the meditation arts. But before any luxuries of theory, theology, and practice, we had to work. No task was too menial nor too advanced for anyone. We took our assignments and pulled our weight with no questions or complaints. At first, I was given the task of polishing the brass fittings around the huge wooden doors at the entrance and along the ground floor. One day, having climbed a ladder to reach the top,

DOI: 10.4324/9781003223603-16

I slipped and found myself hanging precariously from a ledge, by my fingernails, as I later described it. Instantly, before I could muster a scream, a solid wall of sound materialized beneath me and there stood Muhan and Anicca, making no move to physically assist me, but chanting hard at me from the very insides of their bones. I can never do justice to the memory in words but I felt myself lifted, supported, and in absolutely no danger of a fall. Somehow, I clambered to a safe position and then down to stand on the floor, utterly astonished. "What did you do?" I asked, "Because that defies logic!" Muhan and Anicca simply grinned at me and went on about their own business but when they grew impatient with my relentless questions about sound-spells; about how frequency, resonance, magic, and intention could literally manifest as a wall of sound, they had me assigned to the Evening Bell. This was for my phenomenological experience of sound as sound should properly be used, and another period of rapid transformation for me.

To fully contextualize the purpose of the temple bells, this has been written of the Morning Bell:

> The magnificent sound of the temple bell shakes the dawn and awakens all living creatures from a dream world. As the brilliant morning sun reddens the eastern horizon, wake up and listen to this bell. Its clarity sings of eternity and infinity, and it resounds endlessly throughout the universe...
>
> People of all races the young and the old, children and adults, males and females, the rich and the poor all join together in praise at the sound of this bell. When this bell resounds, all oppositions, all hostilities, all conflicts disappear. We all find our pure, fundamental nature, and we all embrace one another as a family.
>
> Listen to the sound of this bell. As it reverberates, the wooden roadside totems sing and people who are as cold as stone come to life. Everything in the immense universe moves happily at the sound of this bell, so happily that "heaven" and "paradise" become embarrassing terms. If you can't hear this sacred sound, it's because you are deaf with desire and greed. Rid yourself of these temporal cravings, and listen to this eternal sound.
>
> (2016, http://www.buddhism.org/listen-to-the-eternal-sound-of-the-bell/)

Now, Sunim had assigned me to sound the Evening Bell with a book of instructions, including diagrams on how the bell should be engaged and lyrics for the accompanying chant. The pallet must be brought into relationship with the bell, he explained, as unity and harmony are sought between violin and bow or archer and arrow. The bell is thus not *hit* with the pallet or hammer, but it *meets* with the bell at a certain angle, in a certain place, with varying degrees of heaviness and bounce, the aim being to facilitate the sacred union between liturgical instruments and make the instrument and the artist one. Sumin also instructed me in the primary purpose of the Evening Bell, that being to put all sentient beings to sleep with peace in their souls.

Psychoacoustics

Psychophysics is the branch of psychology that deals with relationships between physical stimuli, sensory systems, and mental phenomena. Psychoacoustics is a branch of psychophysics; the branch of science which studies psychological responses associated with sound. This relatively new field, emerging in the late 1800s, had an initial aim to help the development of communications. It would answer such questions as how our bodies receive sound depending upon environmental and cognitive contexts, and how our brains interpret the sounds that we hear. For example, physiological factors like ear shape and size, bone weight and density and the resonance of skulls, all affect how we hear as individuals. Our psychology then processes the meaning of the sounds we hear, decoding source and intent. Some psychoacoustic indicators include tone, pitch, timbre, loudness, roughness, and sharpness.

In the field of engineering, mathematical and computational techniques gauge how sound will be experienced in the design of cars, amusement parks, bicycle bells, sirens, and so on. On a pedestrian level, if we are at a restaurant and hear dishes break, we make instant meaning of that; it is not a threat. However, if we are awoken from sleep in the middle of the night by the same sound of breaking dishes, we are likely to sit bolt upright, hearts racing, experiencing sudden, acute fear.

In the field of music, studies in psychoacoustics began well before the 1800s. In the time of Pythagoras, 6th century B.C., Pythagoreans were fascinated with music and the consonance or dissonance produced by the instruments that were popular then: the flute, the lyre, and the tympanum. The study of sound has continued since then in many different directions.

Skipping past history of psychoacoustics, which is equally as fascinating as it is too long and complex to discuss in this context, I jump ahead to Oliver Sacks (1933–2015), British neurologist and best-selling author, nicknamed "The Explorer of the Brain" and "The Poet Laureate of Medicine". Sacks is best known for writing about syndromes like Tourettes, Aspergers, Autism, and Schizophrenia in a manner that humanized and de-mystified his patients. Following his Soviet mentor, the founder of neuropsychology, A.R. Luria, one of the areas on which Sacks focused on the relationship between music and the brain. One of his several books, Musicophilia (2008), was dedicated to this.

Music is now increasingly used in the care and therapy of the mentally and emotionally impaired. As Kathy Evans wrote of her work with autism, art therapy develops a special communicative relationship between therapist and patient, and it is through this that the inner life of individuals in therapy can be explored. In traditional cultures, even where practitioners do not speak the language of Western science, music has always been applied in distinctly therapeutic ways. Different rhythmic or overtone patterns can modify heartbeat and breath frequency, influence adrenalin or stress levels, modify behavior, and bring about the integration of a disordered personality. As mentioned in the chapter on Maddinks and her use of traditional, ritual music and dance as well as in the chapter on Vladimir where we speak of Dionysus and the Jab Jab, a great many diverse, culture-specific applications of music therapy have always been in the world. In Kensington Market, Toronto, circa 2005, a veritable constellation of wisdom traditions around sound witnessed Bahira's spectacular breakdown.

As I looked out the windows of the temple's vast second floor, from where I could see a full world of people heading home in the lamplight, I was filled with a sense of sacred responsibility and with tears in my eyes, I hit the bell an almighty whack. The only sound I heard, once the gong stopped reverberating around in my head, was the sound of rage coming from Sunim. I balk at repeating his reprimand here, but suffice to say that I had revealed myself to be in dire need of my own mental stability first, before I could approach the temple bell again.

When, months later, I touched that bell and heard my very teeth sigh as if in gratitude and prayer, I understood. The concept is discussed in many of the world's wisdom traditions, as in Chinese rain-making, the Tao's focus on breath and intention, and the harmonies between body-mind and heaven-earth, but in short the ancient practices speak to the necessity of experiencing your own true self before setting out to heal the world.

Bahira

When Bahira hit her own bell that fated evening, so to speak; when her soul was ripped from her body by a predator and she let out a sound that personified what she believed was her spiritual death, all sentient beings in Kensington Market who heard her, lifted their heads and trembled.

Bahira was a 13-year-old girl, the only child of a loving family whose lives revolved around a fundamentalist religious community. Bahira was happy in every sense of the word. She soaked up the love of her parents and extended family members, did extremely well at school and with all of her extra-curricular activities, and loved Jesus Christ. Bahira glowed from within and church elders whispered that they could virtually *see* her aura, so pure and resplendent it was. She followed all of the rules set out by her community of faith and although now in full puberty and very attractive to boys and men, she observed the expectation of no sex before marriage and prided herself in tending her body as the temple of her living God.

When Bahira's family welcomed a young male cousin, three years Bahira's senior, to come to stay in their home whilst attending college, he raped Bahira, and she instantly shattered. Worse, he made her pregnant and her parents, equally as shattered as Bahira was, arranged for a quick termination of the pregnancy. Bahira fell headfirst into an immense, terrifying madness. She believed herself expelled from the presence of God and the possibility of Heaven, through no fault of her own.

According to her religion, as with all three Abrahamic religions and Sunim's instructions on sounding the evening bell from the Zen Buddhist temple on the other side of the street, if one goes to sleep in a good way, being calm and in remembrance of God, God sends angels to sit at one's head while you sleep so if you die during the night, your soul will be taken directly heavenward. Sufism also teaches that God takes the soul of His servant and replaces it with a new form of life with and in Himself.

But now Bahira was beset by nightmares and flashbacks that molested her sleep and threw her awake several times a night, choking violently and sweating through her sheets. (Years later, when she was diagnosed with obstructive sleep apnea among other illnesses "with no medical cause", she had no doubt of the origin of her trouble). "No part of the sin was mine" she often said, "God abandoned me and took with him all of his angels, leaving me to face hell alone". Bahira began a journey through the valley of the shadow, slipping into residence within a ghostly, dissonant realm where she no longer believed in a future, whether on earth or in the hereafter. She felt herself to be ghostly; without substance, an unstable, ephemeral non-present entity, neither dead nor alive. Worst, she no longer felt the nearness of her God, nor believed in justice. Yet she became terrified of death because now she was sure that Heaven was denied her, while Hell was waiting to consume her in eternal flames. One can well imagine Nietzsche's cry, "God is dead. The God of Love is dead!" Bahira had no ontological status, as Derrida would say, nor could she situate herself within an eschatological framework; hence her occupying the space of hauntology. Bahira lived without expectation, promise, or commitment in a liminal space between life and death.

The professionals into whose hands she first fell were medical and psychiatric doctors, as Bahira's terror of hellfire and death led her toward hypochondria, panic attacks, body dysmorphia, and a diagnosis of psychosis. But despite their administrations, Bahira's personality split into two parts. One part of her felt lost and alone, but another part somehow refused to give up, struggling to locate and befriend the indestructible self that remained hovering, just always out of reach.

Bahira's selves began to call to and converse with each other while just outside her bedroom, her mother sat on the floor, leaning into the door, listening to the cries and answers. "Come on girl!" She whispered into her handkerchief. "You can do it! Come on!" And Dad paced up and down, tears flowing from his eyes. When Bahira railed most loudly at her shadows, her mother wailed more loudly still. With her precious child battling the demons of the underworld, she screamed in accompaniment at the furthest extent of her lungs, petitioning God Almighty to save her child's soul. Neighbors listening said they heard the sound of the Zulu war chant, others argued that it was more of a full tribe of Maori performing Haka. Freud may have referred to this as "hieroglyphic" speech. But neighbors agreed that the more spine-chilling sound by far came from the mother not the child, as she crouched outside that bedroom door, keeping pace. "Mummy is holding you with two hands! Mummy will never let you go! I have you in two hands!" Her husband fell to his knees, put his arms around himself and rocked and cried. Too much to bear. Too much. Too much. Somebody help.

Another neighbor on the far side of Bellevue Square barely caught the edge of Bahira's sound at the weft of the evening breeze and turned toward the vibration to feel it better. His heart dropped when he made it out more clearly. Bahira's anguish was traveling miles. "Babylon", he whispered under his breath. "Babylon". He pulled his drum tighter into the space between his thighs and put hands to skin. He also had medicinal purposes, and in this gathering place, Rasta sent up his song for peaceful sleep and for healing.

Then a new, third thing entered. It was a new feminine energy in the form of a psychotherapist from South America, trained and licensed in Toronto. She had the slanted eyes of the indigenous people who have traversed that continent for thousands of years. She arrived on the breeze carrying a Egyptian Ney flute and without a word, sat on the floor outside of Bahira's door, beside Mum and Dad. With effortless grace, she began to play. Somewhere deep inside the shattered consciousness of Bahira, the child heard the flute and began to dream that she was whirling, like angels. Her mind emptied, but no longer did she feel alone. The flute music provided a ladder upon which she felt she could steadily climb, though the destination remained hidden among clouds.

A force, or a barakah; a divine energy, circulated the space on the wings of this Ney. In Islam, barakah means blessing or a blessing power that begins with God (thus having an ontological hierarchy) and comes to flow between people, places, materials, and actions on a shared plane. Sufi practitioners believe that this force (not a feeling, not a bliss, but a force) can alter the condition of bodies here on our plane. This is one reason why the Qu'ran is meant to be recited or *heard*, and not silently read, as those of the faith believe that the sound of the message itself carries a force of blessings. Oliver Sacks, neurologist and author, often wrote of his success with music for patients who could not be reached by the standard psychiatric methods, such as patients with schizophrenia and autism. He remarked that music occupies far more of our brain than language does.

> Music can lift us out of depression or move us to tears – it is a remedy, a tonic, orange juice for the ear. But for many neurological patients, music is even more – it can provide access, even when no medication can, to movement, to speech, to life. Furthermore, music is not a luxury, but a necessity.
>
> (Sacks, 2008)

Sufism, like some of the yogic practices, identifies the localization of thought in the body-mind, and Paul Stoller carried this forward into group consciousness when he wrote of his ethnographic fieldwork. "Recognition of multisensorial perception leads to a more embodied, radically phenomenological approach ... a more rigorous framework of the analysis of culture-in-society" (Stoller, 1995, p. 16). Similarly, Jung wrote of coming into connection with the *numen*, a transcendental dimension where the original spirit informing all life dwells, and in this space, bridges between the polarities that split us – the conscious and unconscious, psyche and matter, man and nature – may be built, and we may heal. Music is often the medium.

Coming full circle, Martin-Baro writes of the ongoing dilemma between psychology and religious anthropology. With reference to the psychologies that emerged from laboratories and scientism, religious people were quick to label it "rat psychology" as opposed to a psychology of the soul. This type of laboratory-based psychology was seen as dangerous to religious faith. Similarly, arguments continue to exist between psychologies that are reactionary rather than progressive, humanistic rather than materialistic, and so on. In Martin-Baro's way of thinking, each practitioner should know sufficiently about these diverse theories and approaches to be able to choose the one that best serves each individual client and their unique treatment plan. Speaking of his own people, Martin-Baro called for a psychology that focused on the client and not on the practitioners or their institutions. He called for a scientific commitment to find, and more important, do, what is true for our Latin American people. Psychology, he believed, could do even more than rid people of their individual suffering, but also make a substantial contribution to the evolution of our nations. Jung's theories on cultural complexes had the specific aim of analyzing the trajectory between individual experience and mass manifestations of these complexes in political and military as well as religious communities. In the discipline of psychohistory, theorists are in the thick of discussions about how the individual personality lends itself to cultural traits that perpetuate war-mongering on a larger scale than ever seen before, and at the Jungian Society of Montreal, Tom Singer is currently holding talks on "Cultural Complexes in our times: The Russian/Ukraine war and other cases".

In the case of Bahira, this new South American practitioner had not been formally contracted but had heard of the patient's psychotic break in the village of Kensington, and she showed up to volunteer her time, without a word.

Archetypal Psychotherapy

A psychotherapist, like an archer, trains how to shoot in all circumstances. The therapist cannot always choose the mental terrain or know in advance whether the ground will be dangerous, but she comes prepared for unfavorable situations. This is the energy of Artemis, as I discussed before, and Isabel Allende has written "Artemis is arising in popular culture as a new source of strength, power and integrity. She is the protector of life, the activist who never gives up, the idealistic heroine who cannot be subdued".

This journey takes up the entirety of a lifetime and as I learned from Sunim, it can only be undertaken with peace in one's soul. As Frankl wrote, "A psychotherapist is continually concerned with spiritual existence in terms of freedom and responsibility, and with marshaling it against the psycho-physical facticity that the patient is prone to accept as (her) fate" (Frankl, 2000, p. 33) Or, to quote from Romme and Escher, "the art of therapy is to keep an open mind because there is so much variation between people who suffer from an emotion. Therapy requires using bits and pieces from many theories and using them at the moment when the person is motivated to consider ideas" (p. 2)

"Bahira is calling for something that she knows she has in her own soul", the therapist told Bahira's parents. "I will simply sit with her while she does this work in her own way".

"You mean to say you will leave her to go mad?"

The therapist smiled quietly. "You might say so, but I believe she will come back".

"She feels she has lost her soul", she explained, tilting her head toward the wind coming in off Lake Ontario in the distance. "This is not unusual when young people are violated, but the thread remains. It is my job to hold the thread fast for her, as she cannot do it for herself right now. But she will pick it up herself again. Patience".

While friends and family are usually very grateful for periods of time when a distressed person's psychosis seems to be kept under control, subdued, medicated, or otherwise suppressed, Jung regards this period of suppression as unfortunate. For him, it is important to face mental health breaks squarely, openly, and patiently as Bahira's therapist was leading her to do. In this way, one can directly observe what is arising in the psyche and be sure of what tools, instruments, and routes the healing should take.

Indigenous people believe that a soul can become separated from its body, or dis-embodied, under conditions of grief, anger, or fear. The Hmong people of Laos, for example, additionally believe that "a baby's soul may wander away drawn by bright colors, sweet sounds or fragrant smells, or … if the baby is sad, lonely or insufficiently loved by its parents" (Fadiman, 1997). To guard against the latter, elaborate rituals are performed at a child's birth in which a child's parents promise to love him or her. In any event, as astronomical rates of child abuse illustrate that promises from parents to love their babies are not always made, or not kept, a very advanced psychology has developed over time to help the unloved and the violated. Whether one calls it soul loss, spirit possession or psychosis, the patient is suffering the same and needs some manner of help.

Incidentally, as with every perpetrator in this book except Vladimir's, Bahira's abuser was never brought to justice nor was he reprimanded much. Being from the same fundamentalist religious family and community as Bahira, the internal supervisory mechanisms among the church elders convinced Bahira's family not to report him and ruin the reputation and future of the male child. The tendency of cultures to silence perpetrators is often amplified the more closed and religious the society is and in fact, it is known that some religious preferences provide leeway for sex offenders; a fact that victims in these communities know very well.

So, just like that, the village placed none of its attention on Bahira's teenage rapist, but turned to discussions about religion and its connection with psychosis, perhaps unconsciously finding the abstract, theoretical conversations much more comfortable than the issue of Bahira's spectacular breakdown.

Throughout the social chaos surrounding Bahira and her family so publicly, the psychotherapist remained, sitting cross-legged on the floor, holding space, aiming for sanity. The sound of her Ney continued to pour over Bahira's body like cool river water; like liquid murmurs; like indigo milk. Finally, Bahira began to feel clean.

Bahira's case was passed on to me after she had worked with that therapist for some time and had been stabilized by her. It now fell to me to provide the easier part, a course of cognitive behavioral and depth therapies that would help with flashbacks, nightmares, anxiety attacks, and re-building healthy relationships within the community, particularly with males.

I entered the home at precisely the moment when Bahira's parents were bidding the therapist goodbye and I heard the Mum say, "We have been calling you 'Miss' all this time, and I am embarrassed to say we still don't know your first name. What is your name?" The therapist turned around to face Bahira's parents and myself at the same time, and my mouth fell open.

"My name is Yara", she said.

We embraced each other for a long time, just taking each other in, arms wrapped tightly around, forehead to forehead. It had been at least 15 years since I had seen her, but this is a moment I will remember forever. How that beautiful child had grown, and as she stepped off the porch in the warm Toronto night, Ney flute underarm, I saw her tilt her head in that old familiar way, listening for her sound of her father's voice.

References

Fadiman, A. (1997). *The Spirit Catches You, and You Fall Down*. Farrar, Strauss and Giroux.

Frankl, V. (2000). *Man's Search for Ultimate Meaning*. Perseus Publishing.

Stoller, P. (1995). *Embodying Colonial Memories: Spirit Possession, Power and the Hauka in West Africa*. Routledge.

Sacks, O. (2008) Musicophilia: Tales of Music and the Brain, Vintage Canada.

Index